Praise for *The Medical Marijuana Handbook*

The medical uses of marijuana are changing the lives of thousands of individuals and these applications will continue to expand. Norma Eckroate's *The Medical Marijuana Handbook* sheds much-needed light on this rapidly evolving field.

> **Larry Dossey, MD,** author of *ONE MIND: How Our Individual Mind Is Part of a Greater Consciousness and Why It Matters*

The Medical Marijuana Handbook provides an in-depth and personal look into one of the leading untapped resources in modern medicine. In her wonderful book, Norma Eckroate provides insights as both a patient and a researcher on the history of cannabis, its benefits and applications, and dosing. She also explains why cannabis is one of the most beneficial medicines available today because of the unique and holistic ways that it heals. I highly recommend this book to anyone who is on a healing journey.

> **John Hicks, MD,** author of *The Medicinal Power of Cannabis: Using a Natural Herb to Heal Arthritis, Nausea, Pain, and Other Ailments*

The Medical Marijuana Handbook is a must read for anyone who wonders if cannabis might help them. In this excellent book, Norma Eckroate provides us with a layperson's primer on the science behind cannabis. She also explains her own journey with the herb, including her initial reluctance to tell anyone she was "using" it and her great surprise at the degree to which it almost immediately quelled her symptoms. This book is chock-full of practical information – and I especially appreciate Eckroate's holistic perspectives and her body-mind-spirit approach.

> **Ronit Lami, PhD,** psychologist, speaker, and contributing author, *Roadmap to Success*

Eckroate tackles the confusion of the newly emerging medical marijuana arena flawlessly. She is concise but thorough, scholarly yet practical. For anyone who is a medical marijuana patient, this book answers all your questions. Eckroate writes from personal experience in a clear and friendly tone. Her heart-felt aim is to leave the reader well-informed and reassured. And she succeeds brilliantly. You will treasure this book.

Joan Bello, author of *The Benefits of Marijuana* and
The Yoga of Marijuana

In this comprehensive book, Eckroate shares practical knowledge and skillfully addresses the many questions and issues that arise for medical marijuana patients, literally "holding their hands." An accomplished writer and researcher in the alternative health care field, Eckroate also shares her own personal quest as a patient for whom marijuana has vastly improved the quality of her life. Highly recommended for anyone considering the use of this kind herb, with its remarkable healing powers, to treat any medical condition regardless of one's past experience with it.

David Hoye, author of *Cannabis Chemotherapy*

The

MEDICAL

MARIJUANA

HANDBOOK

A Patient's Guide to Holistic Healing with Cannabis

Norma Eckroate

Disclaimer

This book details the author's personal experiences with and opinions about medical marijuana. The author is not a healthcare provider.

The author and publisher are providing this book and its contents on an "as is" basis and make no representations or warranties of any kind with respect to this book or its contents. The author and publisher disclaim all such representations and warranties, including for example warranties of merchantability and healthcare for a particular purpose. In addition, the author and publisher do not represent or warrant that the information accessible via this book is accurate, complete or current.

The statements made about products and services have not been evaluated by the U.S. Food and Drug Administration. They are not intended to diagnose, treat, cure, or prevent any condition or disease. Please consult with your own physician or healthcare specialist regarding the suggestions and recommendations made in this book.

Except as specifically stated in this book, neither the author or publisher, nor any authors, contributors, or other representatives will be liable for damages arising out of or in connection with the use of this book. This is a comprehensive limitation of liability that applies to all damages of any kind, including (without limitation) compensatory; direct, indirect or consequential damages; loss of data, income or profit; loss of or damage to property and claims of third parties.

You understand that this book is not intended as a substitute for consultation with a licensed healthcare practitioner, such as your physician. Before you begin any healthcare program, or change your lifestyle in any way, you will consult your physician or other licensed healthcare practitioner to ensure that you are in good health and that the examples contained in this book will not harm you.

This book provides content related to topics of physical and/or mental health issues. As such, use of this book implies your acceptance of this disclaimer.

Dedication

This book is dedicated to the many leading edge pioneers who have worked tirelessly for decades—and, in many cases, sacrificed greatly—to reestablish marijuana as the preeminent healing medicine that it had been for thousands of years. They are generous, intelligent, kind people who have been driven to help those who desperately need this healing herb. I appreciate all of them, including many whose names we will never know. Medical professionals who have led the way include Dr. Lester Grinspoon, Dr. Tod H. Mikuriya, Dr. Uwe Blesching, Dr. Allan Frankel, Dr. Jeffrey C. Raber, and Dr. William Courtney, to name just a few. And many ordinary citizens have played important roles too, including Jack Herer, Rick Simpson, Dennis Peron, "Brownie Mary" Rathbun, and Terence Hallinan, former District Attorney of San Francisco.

I also dedicate this book to the wonderful doctors and other health professionals who have treated me over the last decade or so, especially Dr. Joseph Sciabbarrasi, Dr. Ronald Andiman, Dr. Victoria Wexley, Dr. John Hicks, and Dean Murray. I am extremely appreciative of these kind, caring, and leading edge healers who have helped immensely on my path to greater well-being.

Finally, this book is dedicated to my fellow medical marijuana patients. May you heal, prosper, and be well!

Acknowledgements

My deep appreciation goes to all of those who have cheered me on in the two-and-a-half year journey of writing this book. It feels that I have an almost endless number of loving supporters—far too many to list them all here. However, I must single out some whose support has been over-the-top. First, I thank Cara Newell, Karen Lorre, and Carilyn Davidson, soul sisters whose love and support have been epic and life-affirming. Also, I am extremely appreciative to the leading edge friends who have played important roles in my cannabis journey. They include Kathy Eldon and Claire Humphrey, wise women who are dedicated to being beneficial presences on this planet and who connected me with others who contributed greatly to this venture; Mary Ann and David Hoye, whose love and support and friendship are boundless and who gave me valuable input on more drafts of this book than I can recall; Patrick Lang and Tina Hulett, kind and loving souls whose comments on drafts were immensely helpful and whose friendship is invaluable; Scotty Meyler, a generous and loving friend who connected me with John Hicks, MD and Betsy Hicks; and, finally the aforementioned Hickses, for their generous supportiveness and input.

I also want to thank the many generous friends and associates who read early drafts of this manuscript and gave me valuable input, including Rosemary Ahern; Margaret Laspino; Cara Newell; Anastasios Nestoras, PhD; Kris Taylor; Anitra Frazier; Mary L. Brennan, DVM; Jan Leuken; Stephen McCamman; Arita Trahan; Elizabeth Reyes, PhD; Elizabeth Torres, PsyD; Cecelia Pizzolo, PhD; Sandy Weir, RN; Jerry V. Teplitz, PhD; and Annaleah and Joshua Atkinson.

My appreciation for my publishing "team" is boundless: Francis Sporer for his awesome cover design; Julie Isaac for her savvy promotional insights and editing talent; and Melissa Knight for her great marketing proposals and cheerleading. I am also very appreciative of the professionalism and talent of everyone at BookLocker!

Contents

Important

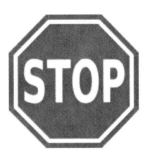

Please Read This First!

Many patients extol the healing and symptom relief of medical marijuana.

However, if you elect to use marijuana as a medicine, it is wise to consider other medicines and treatment options alongside it that might prove effective or, in some cases, even critical to your recovery.

I also urge you to tap into the holistic perspective that body, mind, and spirit are all involved with the healing process.

Start with a VERY SMALL Dose

It is important to start with a very, very, very small dose of cannabis medicine and increase your dosage slowly, UNLESS:

1) You are taking one of the cannabis products that do NOT cause a psychoactive "high" or "stoned" feeling; OR

2) You have developed a tolerance to cannabis through prior use.

If you take too much of a cannabis product that causes psychoactivity, you may have to take a very long nap or even sleep it off for a day or longer. It is strongly advised that you consult a medical marijuana health professional about your product choices and dosage.

A Note About Terminology

It would be helpful if all medical marijuana experts used the exact same terminology; however, that's not the case at this point in time. Here's some clarification on a few terms:

- *Is it marijuana or cannabis?*
  I use the words **marijuana** and **cannabis** inter-changeably. Marijuana goes by a number of names, including cannabis and hemp, as well as many slang terms, including weed, pot, grass, hash, Mary Jane, and ganja. Actually, marijuana is a slang term too, since *cannabis* is the scientific name for this herb. Even though I use both words, I use the word cannabis more often since that's the real name.

- *Is "hemp" the same as cannabis?*
  The term *hemp* has different meanings to different people. In some parts of the world, the word *hemp* is often used for strains of cannabis that are medicinal. In the United States, *hemp* generally refers to varieties of the cannabis plant that are used in making nutritional supplements or industrial products, including some cannabis medicines that are made from strains of the plant that are extremely low in THC (tetrahydrocannabinol), the chemical that causes psychoactivity, and high in CBD (cannabidiol), a chemical that is considered to have more healing benefits for some conditions.

- ***What is "cannabis oil"?***
  When I refer to *cannabis oil*, I'm referring to concentrated medicinal cannabis products that are manufactured through an extraction process. As I explain in Chapters 3 and 18, different manufacturers use different names for this type of oil.

- ***What does psychoactivity mean?***
  Psychoactivity is a term used to describe an alteration in a person's mood or perception when a substance, such as the chemical THC in marijuana, travels through the bloodstream and into the brain. These alterations can include positive experiences, such as euphoric feelings, relaxation, increased alertness, and an altered sense of time and space—or, for those who take extremely high doses or have a very low tolerance level, negative experiences, such as hallucinations, paranoia, anxiety, or impaired memory. **As explained in this book, some forms of cannabis are now available that produce *little* or *NO* psychoactivity.**

About Chronic Pain

Medical cannabis can help to quell pain, one of the most common symptoms patients deal with. However, did you know that leading edge neuroscientists have found that chronic pain can develop into a disease condition on its own? If you are experiencing long-term pain that is often excruciatingly severe from a condition that should have healed, this new understanding of the reasons for chronic pain—and the solutions for it—might be life-changing for you. Medical marijuana may help in the short-term; however, I urge you to look into this breakthrough understanding in pain as well.

Leading edge doctors and scientists at the forefront of neuroplasticity explain that the extreme level of pain that many patients experience is caused by the "plasticity" of the brain going haywire. As these scientists learn more about the brain's plastic nature—the ability it has to "rewire" itself—they find that many people are suffering from an elevated experience of pain because their brains are literally creating *more* pain. This type of persistent and severe pain, experienced repeatedly over months or years, is called "wind-up pain," "learned pain," or chronic pain syndrome. When this happens, the "pain centers" in the brain can expand and actually hijack surrounding areas—taking over other "cortical real estate"—and causing the elevation in pain.

In a brain that's been hijacked by pain in this way, each of the nine main areas that are designed for processing pain can expand and encompass an area up to five times larger than normal, a fact that is easy to validate with brain scans. When this happens, the areas of the brain that have been hijacked are unable to perform their normal functions as well as they previously did, potentially impacting the ability to deal with tasks such as problem solving, planning, conflict resolution, autobiographical memory, regulating emotions, and relieving pain. Chronic pain often results in a noisy brain, a confused brain, a foggy brain, difficulty with focus and attention, and a constant feeling of being overwhelmed. A "dull" feeling overrides life, and the act of processing a thought or answering a question takes a huge amount of energy. While a patient with this condition may still function fairly well in some of life's arenas, other tasks may feel overwhelming and cause suffering.

The work of experts on this topic has upleveled my life tremendously. I believe anyone who might be dealing with this type of chronic persistent pain will benefit from the leading edge techniques developed by a number of doctors and scientists who are at the forefront of neuroplasticity. I highly suggest you learn more about persistent chronic pain and ways to "take back" any cortical real estate that has been diverted in this way in your own brain by referring to the websites and books of Norman Doidge, MD; Michael H. Moskowitz, MD and his coauthor, Marla D. Golden, DO; Howard Schubiner, MD; John E. Sarno, MD; and Joe Dispenza, DC.

About Product Recommendations

While there are a few exceptions, for the most part, I don't recommend specific products in this book. There are several reasons for this. Each state and jurisdiction around the world that permit the use of medical cannabis has its own regulations. Products that are widely used in one jurisdiction may not be legal in other jurisdictions. Also, I'm hesitant to give product recommendations because a product could provide benefits, such as symptom relief, yet still contain toxins due to being grown on depleted, toxic, or pesticide-laden soil or contain mold, spores, bacteria, viruses, insects, or parasites. Quality control is up to growers and manufacturers who must continually test for both safety and potency. In addition, sometimes a company that produces high-quality products changes management or ownership, which can drastically impact their quality standards.

Introduction

I entered the world of medical marijuana out of desperation. Decades of challenging symptoms from the presumed diagnosis of mild cerebral palsy had beaten me down physically and mentally. Many times, over many years, I thought about how medical marijuana might help. But the craziness around this herb scared me off—until, one day, I finally looked into it. And I'm so glad I did.

In this book I have distilled information that I found helpful in my personal quest to understand the herb, its various forms, and the newly available options in strains and product types. This information is culled and sifted from numerous sources and presented from a layperson's perspective; it is as up-to-date and accurate as possible. My desire is answer your questions, soothe your concerns, and give you the information that you—or a family member or friend—need to better understand it from a holistic perspective so you can effectively use it if that is your choice.

I also share some specifics about the choices I've made, as well as experiences that other patients have shared with me. My focus isn't to give you information on how to roll and smoke a joint, how to use a bong or pipe, recipes for edibles, or how to grow your own marijuana, which is beyond the scope of this book. All of that information is available in books, magazines, and on the Internet. Also, the legalities of medical marijuana are changing so rapidly that getting into those specifics as they relate to countries and states around the world would be fruitless because it would be out of date before this book is published.

Finally, the list of conditions that are now being effectively treated with marijuana is long and exhaustive—and it is constantly being added to; therefore, a list would be out-of-date before it was published. And, anyway, it's best if you do your own research to obtain the most current information possible from experts and from other patients for the condition you're dealing with.

Chapter 1

Welcome to the World of Medical Marijuana

When I first became a medical marijuana patient, I was shocked at how effective it was at quelling challenging symptoms that I've dealt with for years. The results I experienced, from the very first day I took it, were dramatic. I had heard lots of great things about medical marijuana over the years, but I really didn't expect it to be *that* beneficial.

As medical cannabis quickly became my lifeline to greater well-being, I realized that I'd been stuck in stereotypes fostered by decades of slanted and incorrect ideas about this gift from Nature. I started to see it as the amazing herb that so many people have long proclaimed it to be. I was curious about why it was so effective for me and disappointed that I hadn't tried it sooner—so I began to research this much-maligned herb. The more I learned about marijuana, the more I understood how complex—and fascinating and unique—it is. I found myself navigating a confusing maze filled with unfamiliar terminology, numerous types of cannabis products to choose from, and very little specific direction on the best options for me.

Marijuana has been called a sacred herb, a superherb, a Goddess herb, a master herb. As with other herbs and plants, it is imbued with compounds that work together synergistically. However, it is distinguished in the world of botanicals because its many wide-ranging, health-promoting qualities are exceptional. Studies around the world confirm the vast number of beneficial effects that marijuana has on the body and, often, also the mind.

Among the many things I learned is that most of the medicinal strains of cannabis are very different from the strains that recreational users prefer. And that makes sense. The recreational user's goal is generally to achieve the psychoactive "high" or "stoned feeling" that most people associate with it, while—for many medicinal cannabis patients—the high is an unwanted side effect.

My Experience Becoming a Medical Marijuana Patient

As a resident of California with a verified medical need, I could have qualified as a medical marijuana patient when it first became legal in the state in 1996. But, like many others, I hadn't pursued it because the federal government's continued war on this amazing herb scared me away from even trying it. Over those years, many Californians learned the hard way that their state law didn't protect them from seizure of property, arrest and prosecution by the federal government. Many growers, dispensary owners, patients, and parents of patients who are minors ended up in prison, with a criminal record for the rest of their lives. As of this writing, news stories of these "crackdowns," including seizures and arrests, still occur throughout the world, although not nearly as often in some jurisdictions. Thankfully, the situation is improving and cannabis is now available to many patients who have not had access to it in the past.

As I continued to study cannabis as a medicine, I was shocked to learn so much that I didn't know, yet felt I *should* have known. I've written about holistic health and complementary modalities off and on for several decades and thought I knew quite a bit about these topics, including the subject of herbal medicine. My personal health choices have always veered away from pharmaceutical drugs as much

4

as possible, preferring the most natural and holistic treatments to the potential negative side effects that are part and parcel of most pharmaceuticals. At one point in time, I didn't even have a pain reliever like aspirin in my house because I didn't want to take pharmaceutical drugs unless I felt it was needed as a last resort. Then I came to understand that—just as the side effects of a drug are a stress on the body, so is pain.

I had become much less judgmental about pharmaceutical drugs but continued to be cautious, always preferring the natural route when possible. However, over time, as my health condition became much more challenging, I took more and more over-the-counter pain medications to help me sleep at night and got up during the night to take even more when they wore off. I alternated from one type to another to minimize the potential for negative side effects and my doctor frequently did blood tests since some of these drugs can cause serious liver problems.

Eventually, I was referred to a new specialist, who urged me to take a prescription drug to help me sleep at night. I acquiesced because the constant pain and exhaustion were unrelenting. Over time, the doctor added two more drugs to my nightly regimen, all with the goal of a good night's sleep. Combined, the sleeping pill, painkiller, and muscle relaxant led to better sleep than I had experienced in a long, long time. I knew that my doctor was focused on resolving the problems that caused my need for these drugs— seeing them as a short-term solution while she also treated me for sleep apnea and with trigger point injections for muscle spasms and pain. Nevertheless, my doctor and I were both concerned about the addictive qualities of these pharmaceutical drugs.

As with the over-the-counter pain medications, over time, my body became tolerant to the prescription drugs, which had stopped giving me the results I so desperately desired. It got to the point that every night I would wake up after about three hours and have to take more pills in order to get back to sleep. Then I would be awake for an hour or two in the middle of the night, waiting for the new round of drugs to kick in so I could get a bit more sleep before morning.

Every attempt I made to go off even one of these drugs made sleep more elusive. Knowing that I had been on these drugs much longer than my doctor wanted, I treaded gently onto the topic of medical marijuana with her, asking her opinion about whether it might help. I greatly respect her for many reasons, including her integrative approach of combining Western medicine with alternative modalities and treatments. But I didn't have any idea how she'd answer this question and was surprised at her immediate and positive response, almost as if it was she who brought up the subject of medical marijuana instead of me.

My doctor smiled and told me she liked the idea and thought medical marijuana might help. She didn't know much about it but she did know another doctor from whom I could get the official state recommendation—and she even had her staff make an appointment with him for me. Her positive response and encouragement helped open the door to this whole new world and, most importantly, opened the door to less pain and better sleep from the very first night I tried it.

I was thrilled that I was able to replace three pharmaceutical drugs with one little capsule of cannabis extract. And that one little capsule worked *better* than the drugs. The more I studied cannabis, the more I realized that to really understand it, I would have to set aside all of the old negative stereotypes that I had heard all of my life. I searched books and numerous websites and queried people who might be "in the know" for the specific information that would help me understand how it works and why it appears to be so much more efficacious in healing than hundreds of other botanicals that are used around the planet. As I share some rather extraordinary facts about this healing herb, I suggest that you may want to rethink it too. Even if you know a lot about marijuana, so much is changing that there's a good chance that you'll find many new-to-you facts on these pages.

Each Strain of Cannabis Has Unique Healing Benefits

I learned that the hundreds of naturally-produced chemical compounds in cannabis bring balance and harmony to all of the body's systems and that each strain of cannabis acts almost like a different medicine. That's because each strain contains a different ratio or proportion of chemicals based upon its unique genetics and the conditions in which it was grown. Also, because each person's body chemistry is different, there's no guarantee that two patients will find the same cannabis product to be equally efficacious—even if they've been given the same diagnosis and are dealing with the same symptoms.

The world of medical marijuana has been evolving at a fast pace—and stories of cannabis patients finding symptom relief from a variety of illnesses show up in the media frequently these days, each bringing with it great elation. It was about two years ago that I first started hearing about the symptom relief that some patients, including desperately sick young children with seizure disorders, experienced with strains that were newly available. In a way, though, these new strains aren't "new" as much as they are newly reformulated. They are simply attempts by medical cannabis growers and manufacturers to re-create the healing strains that were prevalent and frequently prescribed by doctors until early in the 20th Century.

There are around 400 chemicals found in any cannabis plant; however, many of those chemicals are present in miniscule amounts, while THC and CBD appear in much greater quantities. Among the many newly bred strains that are being specifically created for medical marijuana patients, some are extremely low in the chemical THC and high in the chemical CBD, which are usually the most prominent chemicals in the plant.

While both THC and CBD provide healing qualities, it is the quantity of THC in the strain that most recreational users are interested in because THC causes the psychoactivity and the high or stoned feeling. That's why, over the last seven decades or so of marijuana prohibition, the illegal back-alley trade created strains that were extremely high in THC. In fact, some of them were so high in THC that they contained little to no CBD at all. So these newly available low-THC, high-CBD medical strains that had recently become available in some places are the exact opposite of the THC to CBD ratio that is desired by recreational users.

Hearing about these new low-THC, high-CBD strains, I was anxious to try one. I knew that these new medical strains were bred to contain more healing benefits, and, because I am very sensitive to THC, I was hopeful to find a cannabis product that I could take during the day without experiencing the psychoactivity that made my body wobbly. I didn't expect anything miraculous; I just wanted a product to help quell my symptoms during the day.

I didn't expect the big surprise that occurred when I first started taking a new high-CBD, extremely low-THC capsule. The very next day, my usual morning coughing attach didn't happen. That was a big deal for me. In addition to other symptoms, a chronic debilitating cough had plagued me for 25 years, which a number of doctors had attempted to treat with limited success. At one point, several years earlier, I started taking a nutritional supplement that lessened the frequency of the cough by about fifty percent. However, it was still a daily problem and debilitating when it occurred. So I was truly surprised the day I woke up and didn't cough at all. To be honest, it took a couple more days for me to actually believe my cough had become much less frequent. Since then, when I take THAT particular cannabis product, the cough recurs intermittently—usually when I am overly tired or overly stressed.

When I started taking the high-CBD, low-THC capsules, I had two cannabis products that, combined, helped with my symptoms more than either product by itself. The new high-CBD capsule product seemed to be a miraculous answer for the decades-long chronic cough—but it didn't help with muscle spasms and pain.

That experience opened my eyes and helped me understand the importance of experimenting with different forms and types of cannabis even if you think you're already being helped as much as possible. Remember, different strains have different benefits. That's why it's helpful to do your own research, consult with doctors and other experts who are knowledgeable about cannabis, try new strains and new products, and experiment with dosage in order to get the most healing benefit possible. Since the two products—made from different strains of cannabis and manufactured by different companies—helped me in different ways, I took both on a daily basis. I took a low-THC product during the day and a high-THC product at bedtime.

More recently, I learned about another form of cannabis that gives patients even more options, which is cannabis that's raw. With rare exceptions, raw cannabis does not cause psychoactivity. So that's helpful for people like me who are sensitive to THC, as well as for treating children. However, just like all other strains, what works for one doesn't necessarily work for all. In addition to putting raw cannabis in salads and juicing it, raw cannabis is also made into cannabis oil through a cold-processing method.

Your Brain Produces Its Own Marijuana

I've written about holistic health for over three decades and thought I knew quite a bit about the subject. However, I was in for a surprise when I learned one of the main reasons that scientists believe that cannabis is so healing: **In the 1990s, researchers discovered that there are natural chemical compounds in cannabis that match receptors in the cells of our own bodies. This discovery was so astounding to the scientific world that a 2004 *Scientific American* article was titled "The Brain's**

Own Marijuana" in reference to these chemicals in cannabis.[1]

Many medical and scientific experts believe that it is this link between the chemicals in the plant and those in the cells of our own bodies that makes cannabis so unique, so good at quelling symptoms and, in some cases, effective at bringing healing to health problems in the body and mind. In fact, the cells in our bodies that are a match for the *cannabinoids* in the cannabis plant were named *endocannabinoids*. Because this discovery is still relatively new, at this point in time, most people—and, I dare say, most doctors—do not realize that they are walking around with receptors in the cells of their own bodies that are named after this herb. If you want to check this out, ask a few individuals—and a few doctors—if they can explain the endocannabinoid system to you. Most will probably say, "What is that?"

To date, scientists have identified two subtypes of cannabinoid receptors in our cells, with the likelihood that more subtypes will be discovered in the future. The two that have been identified are:

> **CB1 receptors**: Found mostly in the brain, spinal cord and other parts of the body including the heart, uterus, testis, liver, small intestine and peripheral cells.
>
> **CB2 receptors**: Found mostly on cells of the immune system, including the spleen, T-cells, B-cells and macrophages.[2]

A healthy immune system supports the body's individual cells as they repair or replace themselves when they're damaged. Receptors, which are structures located on the surface of a cell or inside it—such as enzymes, neurotransmitters, or viruses—are a vital part of this "repair or replace" process. They act like receivers and give instructions to the cells to take a specific action, such as dividing, dying and replacing themselves, or allowing a specific substance into or out of the cell. All of these actions are constantly occurring in the body as a process of normal cell function.

Different strains of cannabis target different receptors in the body. In his leading-edge book, *The Biology of Belief*, cellular biologist Dr. Bruce Lipton explains that the receptors in our cells function like antennas that are tuned to respond to specific environmental signals. I find his overview of the ways in which receptors function helpful in understanding the link between the receptors in the cannabis plant and the receptors in the endocannabinoid system in our body's cells. Dr. Lipton says:

> Receptors function as molecular "nano-antennas" tuned to respond to specific environmental signals. Some receptors extend inward from the membrane surface to monitor the internal milieu of the cell. Other receptor proteins extend from the cell's outer surface, monitoring external signals. Like other proteins ... receptors have an inactive and an active shape and shift back and forth between those conformations as their electrical charges are altered. ... Cells possess a uniquely "tuned" receptor protein for every environmental signal that needs to be read.
>
> Some receptors respond to physical signals. One example is an estrogen receptor, which is specifically designed to complement the shape and charge distribution of an estrogen molecule. When estrogen is in its receptor's neighborhood, the estrogen receptor locks on to it, as surely as a magnet picks up paper clips. Once the estrogen receptor and the estrogen molecule bind in a perfect "lock and key" fit, the receptor's electromagnetic charge changes and the protein shifts into its active conformation. Similarly, histamine receptors complement the shape of histamine molecules, and insulin receptors complement the shape of insulin molecules.

Receptor "antennas" can also read vibrational energy fields such as light, sound, and radio frequencies. The antennas on these "energy" receptors vibrate like tuning forks. If an energy vibration in the environment resonates with a receptor's antenna, it will alter the protein's charge, causing the receptor to change shape. ... because receptors can read energy fields, the notion that only physical molecules can impact cell physiology is outmoded. Biological behavior can be controlled by invisible forces, including thought, as well as it can be controlled by physical molecules like penicillin....

Receptor proteins are remarkable, but on their own they do not impact the behavior of the cell. While the receptor provides an awareness of environmental signals, the cell still has to engage in an appropriate, life-sustaining response, that is the venue of the effector proteins.[3]

Until recently, cannabis was the only plant found to be a match for our body's cell receptors, making this herb incredibly unique and special. However, it didn't make sense to me that there would be only one plant on this vast planet that was a match for our human endocannabinoid receptors. So I wasn't surprised to find new research that indicates that chemicals from plants *other than cannabis* also directly interact with CB1 receptors and/or CB2 receptors or have a chemical profile that is similar to the cannabinoids in cannabis. While research on this subject is in its infancy, the herb Echinacea has been found to be a match for some CB1 and CB2 receptors, with other plants also being investigated for their roles in promoting wellness via the human endocannabinoid system.[4] Meanwhile, some new products combine cannabis and other healing botanicals such as Echinacea to increase the effects and curative properties of both herbs.

Later, we will look at the connection between these receptors in the cells and the healing properties of cannabis that make it so powerful in healing bodily conditions.

The Role of Cannabis in Promoting Homeostasis

There's a lot going on in your body simultaneously; it is set up for balance and harmony, with a goal of promoting maximum wellness. The body's constant effort to maintain equilibrium among all of its internal processes and systems is called *homeostasis*, which the *Merriam Webster Dictionary* defines as "the maintenance of relatively stable internal physiological conditions (as body temperature or the pH of blood) in higher animals under fluctuating environmental conditions."5 Early on in my research, I learned that cannabis has healing properties that promote this important function in the body.

As the body pursues optimal harmony and balance through homeostasis, it is constantly in the process of compensating. When one process or system is out of balance, another process or system compensates for the system that is not fully functioning. One example is the body's ability to regulate temperature. As the body gets too hot or too cold, it will compensate to deal with the change in temperature. That's why you sweat on a hot day; it's the body's way of cooling down.

The "repair and replace" mechanism within all of the cells in your body is also part of homeostasis. In fact, in the second that it took you to read the previous sentence, thousands of your cells were automatically repaired or replaced with new cells. The body's intelligence is mind-blowing and its ability to prioritize is what homeostasis is all about.

Imbalances in any of your body's systems throw it off balance and out of whack and require compensating systems to restore balance. For most of us, these compensating mechanisms kick in automatically and keep us healthy, especially when we're young. If we get a cold or flu, our immune system goes to work and we are soon well again. If there's a toxin in the air, the body compensates, handles it, and we don't even know about it because the body is programmed for wellness. It automatically compensates over and over to ensure survival with the very best outcome. That is, unless it's overwhelmed and unable to handle the challenges that come its way, including infections, parasites, and environmental toxins. And, in addition to the tangible challenges that we deal with in the physical world, emotional traumas and negative thinking can also impact the body chemistry in negative ways and impact our health.

So how does homeostasis fit into the scheme of things when the subject is cannabis? Well, anything that helps the body deal with its imbalances will help it get back into homeostasis. While the ratios of the chemical compounds in cannabis vary from strain to strain, scientists have discovered a wide range of positive effects from these healing chemicals, including effects that are anti-inflammatory, anti-epileptic, anti-ischemic, anti-diabetic, anti-psychotic, anti-nausea, anti-spasmodic, antibiotic, anti-anxiety, anti-depressant, anti-proliferative, and anti-neoplastic (inhibiting development of malignant cells).

Even knowing all of this, it took a while for me to understand why cannabis is so significant and powerful, and why its healing properties are utilized by our bodies to such an amazing extent. As you will learn in these chapters, cannabis truly has a special and unique place in the world of botanicals, which is why many doctors and other health professionals are now recommending it to patients.

Most medicinal herbs give us results over a period of time; their action is usually not very fast and we might not feel the beneficial effects for days, weeks, or even months. That's why it's important to give medicinal herbs time to do their work and not give up on them too soon. It's okay that it takes time, because we understand that medicinal herbs heal on a causal basis. One of my mentors recently used the term "softer" to describe the healing we receive from herbs and many other holistic modalities. I like that terminology because experts in herbal medicine tell us that herbs heal on a deeper level than pharmaceuticals, and that does feel softer to me. When we take a medicinal herb that benefits our body, it does so by getting to the root of problems and restoring balance.

While it can take time for a major health issue to be helped, or in some cases, even resolved with cannabis medicine, most patients experience some of its beneficial effects almost immediately, especially if they are astute in noticing their body's responses. For example, you might immediately notice deeper, more relaxed breathing, and more relaxation in the muscles and skeletal system, which can result in better sleep, fewer bathroom visits during the night, improved lung function, and/or greater endurance and stamina. Cannabis can also quickly boost a patient's mental attitude and it's known for giving quick relief to those suffering from nausea or lack of appetite.
*

Chapter 2

A Brief Look at the History and Current Status of Cannabis

In past centuries, cannabis was grown for many different purposes. The United States Constitution was drafted on hemp paper and the sails on ships of that era were made of hemp canvas. (In fact, the word "canvas" is derived from *cannabis*.) Hemp was considered such an important crop that, for a good part of the history of the U.S., all farmers were *required* to grow it.

When marijuana was declared illegal in the 1930s, hemp production was all but shut down in many parts of the world. Now, thankfully, as medical cannabis becomes more available, there is also a resurgence of industrial hemp—used to make paper, rope, wax, resin, cloth, pulp, paint, and even fuel—as well as nutritional food products. Today, the possibilities for new hemp products seem never-ending; one source indicates that there are now 25,000 products that are being made or could be made from this versatile plant.

Hemp is fast growing and ecological. The North American Industrial Hemp Council, Inc. lists some of its many benefits on their website:

- Hemp can be made into fine quality paper. The long fibers in hemp allow such paper to be recycled several times more than wood-based paper.

- Because of its low lignin content, hemp can be pulped using fewer chemicals -than with wood. Its natural brightness can eliminate the need to use chlorine bleach, which means no extremely toxic dioxin being dumped into streams. A kinder and gentler chemistry using hydrogen peroxide rather than chlorine dixoide is possible with hemp fibers.
- Hemp grows well in a variety of climates and soil types. It is naturally resistant to most pests, precluding the need for pesticides. It grows tightly spaced, out-competing any weeds, so herbicides are not necessary. It also leaves a weed-free field for a following crop.
- Hemp can displace cotton which is usually grown with massive amounts of chemicals harmful to people and the environment. 50% of all the world's pesticides are sprayed on cotton.
- Hemp can displace wood fiber and save forests for watershed, wildlife habitat, recreation and oxygen production, carbon sequestration (reduces global warming), and other values.
- Hemp can yield 3-8 dry tons of fiber per acre. This is four times what an average forest can yield.[6]

As a food source and nutritional supplement, hemp is considered to be a superfood for many reasons. It is highly digestible and a great vegetarian source of protein that contains all 20 amino acids, including the nine essential amino acids that our bodies cannot produce, as well as omega-3 and omega-6 fatty acids, which are balanced at the recommended ratio of three to one. In addition to being a nutritious food on its own, hemp seed is also used to make other products such as cooking oil (hemp seed oil), hemp milk, and hemp protein powder. Hemp is also a great feed for animals. Cattle digest hemp more efficiently than other cattle feeds, so they actually require less feed. And hemp seed has been an ingredient in canary song food for ages because it's known to increase the frequency of a canary's songs.

A review of cannabis history in the last century, both as a medicine and as a crop of rich industrial and nutritional diversity, can easily be conducted in numerous books and on a seemingly endless number of websites. It doesn't take a rocket scientist to see the obvious—between its medicinal, industrial, and nutritional potential, this one plant was such a threat to established industries in the 1930s that they colluded to close it down with scare tactics. And they were so good at the scare tactics that, for most of a century, it worked. Instead of focusing on ways to work in concert with Mother Nature, most multi-national companies have, for decades, done much to spoil her, while at the same time, trying—and, too often, succeeding—in patenting some of the components of her gifts so they can "own" them.

We were warned about the dangers of a greedy and powerful military industrial complex by President Dwight Eisenhower. Days before he left office in 1961, his farewell speech included this: "In the councils of government, we must guard against the acquisition of unwarranted influence, whether sought or unsought, by the military-industrial complex. The potential for the disastrous rise of misplaced power exists, and will persist."[7]

Years ago, I learned a very wise teaching that is expressed in various ways by indigenous cultures around the globe: All of the tribe's decisions should be made by considering the impact of those decisions "to the seventh generation in the future." The goal, of course, is that we collectively pass a beautiful and sustainable planet along to future generations by treading lightly and using resources wisely, with the least toxic impact. I believe that big companies can find sustainable, eco-friendly ways to focus their amazing production, marketing, and distribution channels—and still rake in profits.

Contradictory and Confusing Perspectives from the Powers That Be

Like so many others before me, once I had the official paper in my hand in which my state government sanctioned my right to use an ancient healing herb—without too much concern at that point in time of being arrested—I entered the maze. I was a stranger in a strange land. I had many questions: Where do I get the marijuana? What form of marijuana should I take (including smoking, vaporizing, capsules, edibles, suppositories, creams, salves, and other forms)? What strain or type should I chose? How often should I take it? Unless we have a knowledgeable physician or other ally, these are among the questions most of us must answer for ourselves. In this new and somewhat strange world, we are expected to figure out the details and then decide what's right for us as individuals. In fact, as of this writing, doctors in some jurisdictions are not allowed to tell you anything about medical marijuana.

The biggest shock in the U.S. "war" against cannabis is that one branch of the government says cannabis has *no medicinal value* while, at the same time, a different branch of the U.S. federal government patented the cannabinoid, CBD, *for its medicinal value.* One has to be discerning, and at least somewhat knowledgeable, in order to sift through the mounds of dated, inaccurate, and biased information about cannabis that is presented as truth in books and on the Internet. One of the reasons for this glut of outdated, incorrect, and obviously skewed data was presented by Dr. Sanjay Gupta on his CNN special, *Weed.* He reported that there have been over 20,000 studies on cannabis in the last couple of decades; however almost all of them—94 percent—were focused on studying the deleterious effects and harm caused by marijuana, while only six percent of the studies were focused on the benefits.

Clearly, there is a huge amount of evidence that cannabis has great medicinal value for an untold number of illnesses and conditions. But, as of this writing, the government still controls cannabis research in the U.S. and has allowed an extremely limited amount to be done, with most of it focused on *disproving* the medicinal value of marijuana. As a result, most doctors still refuse to recommend it due to the lack of "scientific" evidence of its efficacy.

Anyone who knows how scientific studies are set up understands that it can be challenging to set up a totally unbiased study. If you want to study "deleterious effects and harm from marijuana," that's what you're looking for—and it's likely that you will set up your research to focus on that. On the other hand, if you want to study "benefits from marijuana," you will set up a study to give you data that proves the benefits of the herb. Unfortunately, for most of the last century, the U.S. government rarely looked for anything good about marijuana. The majority of the studies were done by the National Institute of Drug Abuse, a branch of the government that was focused almost exclusively on funding studies that would continue to demonize cannabis as a dangerous drug. Interestingly, some of the very top medical doctors who now promote cannabis as an important medicine were originally involved in research to debunk its medical benefits and were converted when their studies proved its great merits. Within these chapters I quote from some of them.

Most of us have been brainwashed about the evils of "weed" all of our lives. Governments branded it as dangerous and made it illegal. In the U.S., the Justice Department put it on Schedule I of the Controlled Substances Act, which means it has *no medicinal value* and is one of the most dangerous drugs available. The irony is that while some government agencies continue to view cannabis as a dangerous, illegal drug, other government agencies are well aware of its medicinal value. While people were still being thrown into prison for distributing or using marijuana for medicinal purposes, the government continued to run its own medical marijuana program out of the University of Mississippi. That program, which began in 1976, provides free cannabis each month to the patients who are enrolled in it. All these years later, patients who were originally part of this program are still receiving free cannabis *from the United States government.*

In addition to the government's own contradictory marijuana giveaway program, the craziness continued when the United States Department of Health and Human Services obtained a patent on cannabinoids for their antioxidant and neuroprotective properties. Does this make sense—one government agency tells us that cannabis is a dangerous and illegal Schedule I drug, with *no medicinal value*, while another government agency not only acknowledges its medicinal value but also obtains a patent for it? Now how is that possible, you might ask? Isn't it impossible to patent a plant? Apparently the U.S. federal government can do the impossible.

The abstract of U.S. Patent 6,630,507, entitled "Cannabinoids as Antioxidants and Neuroprotectants," tells us exactly what the U.S. Department of Health and Human Services believes to be true about cannabis and its chemical compounds, cannabinoids. It says, in part:

Cannabinoids have been found to have antioxidant properties.... This new found property makes cannabinoids useful in the treatment and prophylaxis of a wide variety of oxidation associated diseases, such as ischemic, age-related, inflammatory and autoimmune diseases. The cannabinoids are found to have particular application as neuroprotectants, for example in limiting neurological damage following ischemic insults, such as stroke and trauma, or in the treatment of neurodegenerative diseases, such as Alzheimer's disease, Parkinson's disease and HIV dementia.[8]

I am also fascinated by the section in the patent entitled, "Detailed Description of Some Specific Embodiments," which discusses more of what this "invention"—in this case, "compounds" found in the herb cannabis—provide to the body:

This invention provides antioxidant compounds and compositions, such as pharmaceutical compositions, that include cannabinoids that act as free radical scavengers for use in prophylaxis and treatment of disease. The invention also includes methods for using the antioxidants in prevention and treatment of pathological conditions such as ischemia (tissue hypoxia), and in subjects who have been exposed to oxidant inducing agents such as cancer chemotherapy, toxins, radiation, or other sources of oxidative stress. The compositions and methods described herein are also used for preventing oxidative damage in transplanted organs, for inhibiting reoxygenation injury following reperfusion of ischemic tissues (for example in heart disease), and for any other condition that is mediated by oxidative or free radical mechanisms of injury. In particular embodiments of the invention, the compounds and compositions are used in the treatment of ischemic cardiovascular and neurovascular conditions, and neurodegenerative diseases. However the present invention can also be used as an antioxidant treatment in non-neurological diseases.[9]

In addition to this patent, a number of other patents have been granted by the U.S. government for the medicinal value of cannabis, including:

- U.S. Patent 8,790,719: Phytocannabinoids in the treatment of cancer
- U.S. Patent 5,538,993: Compounds according to the present invention are characterized by various beneficial properties such as analgesic, anti-emetic, sedative, anti-inflammatory, anti-glaucoma, and neuroprotective activities
- U.S. Patent 6,448,288: Use of Cannabinoid compounds for inhibiting, inducing apoptosis, antitumoral action
- U.S. Patent 4,876,27: Special use in *cases of acute and of chronic pain
- U.S. Patent 7,179,800: Useful for therapy, especially in the treatment of pain, inflammation and autoimmune disease

Clearly the U.S. government knows that cannabis is actually a safe, effective, and relatively inexpensive medicine; not a dangerous drug with no medicinal value, as the Drug Enforcement Administration has classified it for so long.

A New Look at Some Old Stereotypes

Now let's look at a couple of the stereotypes about cannabis—that cannabis causes the "munchies" and that people who use cannabis are "slackers."

The stereotype that cannabis causes the "munchies" and leads to overeating may be true for some people when they take *some cannabis products*. But, again, it depends on the strain and the individual. Some people who are overweight *lose* weight with no effort on medical cannabis, while those who are underweight are often successful in gaining weight.

I've been overweight for most of my life. Even though I'd dropped quite a bit of weight a few years earlier using a nutritional supplement and doing emotional healing work, when I started taking cannabis, I was still overweight and had been stuck on a plateau for a couple of years. For the first six months or so that I took cannabis, I didn't gain or lose weight. But then, after I started taking a high-potency *cannabis oil* product, which is now manufactured under the name Natur-Oil, I started losing weight with no effort at the rate of one to three pounds a month until I had lost about 30 pounds. I know that cannabis can help balance blood sugar levels and I assume that's one of the many ways it has helped in my body. Instead of getting the "munchies" and overeating, cannabis curbed my appetite and my desire for sweets and carbs. I didn't diet, eliminate or limit any foods, or exercise more. I ate whatever I wanted and enjoyed every bite of everything I chose to eat, including sweets and carbs, finding that my body only wanted small amounts of them. That made weight loss easy. I was still rather shocked on those occasions when I didn't want even a small serving of that yummy-looking dessert being offered to me, but the fact that I didn't WANT it and passed on it for that reason felt really good. I've continued on this trajectory and now feel that I'm "eating to live," rather than "living to eat."

My positive experience with weight loss and cannabis isn't everyone's experience. For some people, the munchies seem to be inevitable. If you experience an uncontrollable urge to munch on food when you take cannabis, rather than fret about this side effect, prepare ahead of time and fill your fridge, freezer, and pantry with healthful foods to snack on. Also, you may find that switching to a different cannabis product will eliminate the munchies or, like me, you may even find that you start losing weight.

Another stereotype that's prevalent is that anyone who uses medical cannabis is a slacker who "just wants to get stoned." My experience is that getting high is NOT the preference of most medical marijuana patients. Our goal is not to get high; our goal is to heal. Thankfully, as I mentioned above, for those of us for whom the high is undesirable, newer strains and forms of non-psychoactive cannabis are now available.

Prominent Voices Join the Pro-Medical Cannabis Forces

As more and more people become aware that marijuana is a remarkable and important medicine, the small number of medical experts who have spent years championing it have been joined by some prominent voices. One welcome voice is that of Dr. Sanjay Gupta, a neurosurgeon and medical correspondent for CNN, who has *apologized* for his 2009 article in *Time* magazine entitled "Why I Would Vote No On Pot."

In a 2013 article entitled "Why I Changed My Mind on Weed," Dr. Gupta totally reversed his previous stand against medical marijuana. He now says that cannabis has "very legitimate medical applications" and "sometimes it's the only thing that works." He apologized for the information he shared in the past on this subject, admitting that he was wrong. Dr. Gupta also said, "I was too dismissive of the loud chorus of patients whose symptoms improved on cannabis. ... We have been terribly and systematically misled for nearly 70 years in the United States, and I apologize for my own role in that."[10]

Another prominent voice who has greatly expanded our knowledge is Dr. Lester Grinspoon, Emeritus Professor of Psychiatry at Harvard Medical School, who has been a pioneer in the medical marijuana world for some time and written about it extensively. Dr. Grinspoon brings a welcome sanity to the conversation about the efficacy of cannabis. In a Boston Globe editorial entitled "Marijuana as Wonder Drug," he wrote:

... [marijuana] is extraordinarily safe—safer than most medicines prescribed every day. If marijuana were a new discovery rather than a well-known substance carrying cultural and political baggage, it would be hailed as a wonder drug.[11]

Cannabis Is Efficacious for Many Conditions and Has Been Used Medicinally Since Ancient Times

Cannabis has been cultivated by cultures around the globe and used medicinally for a myriad of purposes since ancient times. These cultures include Egypt, India, China, and Persia, where historical records show that the healers of the day found cannabis to be efficacious for chronic pain, cancer, spasticity, seizure disorders, infectious disease, nausea, and numerous other conditions.

In today's world, the list of the conditions that doctors and patients say have been helped, dramatically improved, or even cured with cannabis gets longer and longer, with more and more websites and television reports proclaiming praise for what it can do to relieve symptoms and heal us. One website includes an exhaustive list of chronic conditions that a pioneering medical cannabis doctor, Tod H. Mikuriya, MD, successfully treated with cannabis over a period of 14 years. The website can be accessed at http://www.canna-centers.com/dr-tods-list.[12]

Because of the longstanding anti-cannabis bias from governments, the truth about this herb has been distorted for most of the past century. Therefore, when you're researching medical cannabis, it is important to consider the source of any information. Those distortions have been fueled by questionable research studies that were clearly biased. That's why any review of previous research studies, as well as anecdotal stories about medical cannabis, often includes a lot of erroneous or outdated information.

Unfortunately, it's likely that a lot of that old information will be out there and will continue to be touted by anti-cannabis "experts" for some time to come. For instance, I visited a website about the eye condition, glaucoma, which warned patients that medical marijuana was *not* an acceptable choice for treating that condition. Interestingly, the article did not dispute the fact that marijuana is known to work well for glaucoma; however, it purported that it would not be possible to take enough marijuana to have a "clinically relevant" impact on the disease. Medical cannabis experts and many patients who tout their successes in treating glaucoma with cannabis totally disagree with that statement.

How sad for glaucoma patients that a seemingly relevant organization that one would expect to be up-to-date with medical science is so blinded to the truth (pun intended); I'm not going to direct you to this website as an example because I hope they soon update it with accurate information about the healing qualities of cannabis.

Whatever your health challenges might be, I encourage you to research how medical cannabis might specifically help you. I hope you'll keep an open mind as you research the subject, and suggest you take the comments of any naysayers with a grain of salt. Also, remember that some websites are biased to a particular point of view, some with a financial incentive. And some simply copy articles from other sites, potentially making it seem that a particular perspective is more widely held than it is.

If, as a medical cannabis patient, you're on your own without a doctor to guide you, I recommend experimenting with different forms and potencies to discover which is the most beneficial for your body. Also, it's helpful to remain open to new options as medical cannabis experts are constantly developing new, more healing strains as well as new types of products. You may also find that an appropriate protocol includes two or more forms of cannabis that you use at different times of the day—or even simultaneously. For example, a person with skin cancer might take cannabis in capsule form and also put plasters of cannabis oil directly on the skin cancer. Or, a person with colon cancer could take cannabis in capsule form, use a vaporizer, and also use cannabis suppositories.

Having more than one product gives you options. It's also okay to take two different products at the same time, such as a capsule and a tincture. The cannabis delivered via the capsule takes an hour or two to get into the system but its benefits last for a longer period of time, while the tincture is absorbed much faster and therefore provides faster relief, but it does not last as long.

Choices in Potency and Dosage

The range of cannabis products available today is vast; some are very low in potency and others, such as the cannabis oil that I previously mentioned, are extremely high in potency. It's nice to have so many options, but it can be difficult to decide among all of them. Certainly, it's advisable to have a health professional guiding you in product selections. However, at this point in time, there are few medical professionals who are qualified—or, in some jurisdictions, legally allowed—to assist us. The idea that a medicine would be prescribed for us without clear directions and guidelines is something that we're not used to. Nevertheless, for most patients, in addition to choosing our own products, we must also learn to *self-titrate*, which means determining our dosage and frequency of administration.

The main goal of many patients is symptom relief; they want cannabis to quiet or relieve their symptoms. If anxiety keeps you awake, if you have asthma, if you experience pain, or if you are dealing with one of a myriad of other bothersome symptoms, using cannabis for symptom relief may be exactly right for you. However, many patients who are dealing with serious conditions that are acute or chronic are focused on cannabis medicine for its therapeutic, healing qualities. Symptom relief is great, but their main desire is to heal the condition altogether or to achieve improvement in that condition, sometimes even beyond that which medical science suggests is possible.

Many, if not most, of the anecdotal stories available in the media about healing from cannabis are from patients who used the most potent forms that are available today, such as cannabis oil in high dosage protocols. As I detail in Chapter 21, the cannabis oil protocol that many patients follow involves increasing the dosage slowly over several weeks until they are taking one gram a day and then maintaining that very high dose for a couple of months.

While some cannabis-savvy doctors encourage the "more is better" approach for their patients and share success stories based on that protocol, others believe that small quantities are actually more effective. The theory behind this low dose regimen is that small quantities do a better job of stimulating the body's internal healing system and, in the end, lead to even better results. A medical doctor who works with many cannabis patients told me that he's seen patients heal from end-stage cancer on a dosage of two small drops of cannabis oil a day. That's equivalent in size to two grains of dry rice, and it's a vastly smaller dose than the much-larger one gram dose that some people take. Clearly, no one really knows what dosage is needed by any particular individual for symptom relief or healing to occur. Every person's body is different and nobody knows exactly what will work for you.

Topical cannabis products have also been heralded by some patients for all-out healing. One YouTube video from a television news show details the "all-out cure" of five malignant tumors in a man's neck through the use of a cannabis balm or ointment.[13] Of course, I can't vouch for the reliability of this TV news report. While I was surprised that this man's healing was attributed to the use of the topical ointment alone, the video doesn't detail the potency of the cannabis balm, how often he applied it, or how long it took for the healing to take place. But is it possible that the healing reported on this video really happened? I believe so.

We'll dig deeper into various issues related to potency and dosage in future chapters.

Asking the Right Questions

As we approach a tipping point in the modern history of medical cannabis, some experts in this field have been researching, growing, and/or manufacturing products for many years, while others are fairly new to this booming industry. In many cases, these experts are self-educated, having gotten into this business because of their own dire healing needs or those of friends or family members.

The cannabis business owners that I've met are very concerned about providing help to patients. They have taken on great responsibilities, knowing that some patients are facing life or death decisions and others are dealing with quality of life issues. One of these medical cannabis pioneers, Patrick Lang, explained his perspective to me this way, "In the widespread absence of clinical research we—as cannabis patients—are doing our own research. Our facts and theories on cannabinoids come from on-the-job training, individual research, personal experience, educated guesses, and empirical data—in the rare places that it exists."[14]

I am not a medical professional or a scientist; I am simply a writer, a researcher, a spiritual counselor, and a seeker of truth. While healing often requires specific treatments and products, from a holistic, mind-body-spirit perspective, it also involves tapping into the inner wisdom that's always available to our bodies and our consciousness.

I sincerely hope your medical cannabis journey will be easier because of the information on these pages and that it will help speed you on your way to greater wellness. No matter what history you may have with marijuana, pro or con, or what you think you know about it, please put aside any notions or biases for a little while as we continue to explore this sometimes miraculous herb.

Chapter 3

New Options in Medical Marijuana Products Provide Even More Healing Potential

Exciting new options for medical marijuana patients have unfolded in this era, which many are calling the "green rush." Scientific research (mostly outside of the U.S.), anecdotal stories from patients, and discoveries on the news and on the web continuously confirm an increasing number of health benefits from ingesting cannabis. The lives of many patients, some of whom are very young children, have been literally transformed by new strains, new processing methods, new product choices, and new ways to ingest cannabis. After two-and-a-half years of research, I can tell you that many patients—who have dealt with a wide range of physical and mental health problems—say, "Cannabis gave me my life back."

The laws are changing in states and countries around the globe, allowing more and more people to legally access this amazingly healing herb. As the paradigm shifts to greater mainstream acceptance of medical cannabis, both patients and entrepreneurs have stepped into a bold new world in which cannabis is appreciated and honored instead of being misrepresented, defiled, altered, distorted, and debased.

More and more new research studies have been done around the world. And many of them show that cannabis doesn't just quell symptoms; in some cases it also has healing benefits. In the long term, the possibility that cannabis medicine might limit or delay the progression of a health issue and potentially even heal it gives me and other patients great relief. In fact, there's reason to believe that almost any patient could be helped by it:

- **Patients with acute health conditions that are life threatening**.
  Cannabis has been shown to provide symptom relief for many patients and, for some, actual improvement in severe life-threatening health challenges.
- **Patients with chronic health issues.**
  Many patients find that symptoms of chronic health concerns are quelled by cannabis, without the negative side effects of other medications.
- **Patients with sporadic health issues or injuries**.
  Cannabis is also found to be efficacious for many common symptoms, such as pain, anxiety, difficulty sleeping, nausea, etc.
- **Health-conscious individuals who want to stimulate their body's internal healing system with a regular maintenance dose of cannabis.**
  Cannabis helps modulate or balance every human physiological system, including regulating immunity, inflammation, neurotoxicity, blood pressure, appetite, gastrointestinal function, and intraocular pressure. Therefore, many health-conscious individuals desire a small maintenance dose of medical cannabis to promote health and well-being.

In this chapter, we'll look at some of the categories of cannabis products that are popular with patients today. But first, I want to address the question of how much faith we should put into patients' anecdotal success stories.

Are Anecdotal Reports About Patient Successes a Reason to Try Cannabis?

As I heard more and more stories of individuals who proclaimed that cannabis healed them from challenging or even life threatening conditions, I realized that relief of symptoms was only the tip of the iceberg in terms of its potential benefits. These stories of people saying that they have been cured are considered "anecdotal" to most experts, who say they are not to be relied upon as accurate or trustworthy. But since very few patients are prescribed cannabis by their primary care physicians, that means anecdotal reports about the efficacy of cannabis are rarely—in fact, *almost never*—considered viable. Even when major symptoms are relieved or outright healing occurs, without the strict protocol of clinical scientific studies, officially, it just doesn't count as far as they're concerned. Unless a patient is part of a controlled study or being given a medication or treatment by their doctor, positive results are not given any merit by most medical professionals. And, of course, that does make sense to a certain degree.

Without standards and controls, who knows what other factors might have influenced the patient and led to improvement in a condition? But does that mean we should totally dismiss the fact that numerous people report phenomenal healing with cannabis, including reported healings of end-stage cancers and improvement in severe seizure disorders? At what point will the countless anecdotal stories of patients being healed be given merit and, at the very least, be studied so that other patients may benefit, especially when all other options have failed or produced debilitating side effects?

Unfortunately, in the case of cannabis, valid studies that are focused on the healing efficacy of the herb are few and far between. As of this writing, in the U.S., the government controls the studies and it has allowed very few new studies to be conducted. Much of the current research that is propelling our scientific understanding of this herb's healing benefits is currently being done outside the U.S., with Israel, Spain, and Uruguay as leading edge examples.

Harvard psychiatrist Dr. Lester Grinspoon, whom I quoted earlier, is the author of two books written decades ago on this subject, *Marihuana Reconsidered* and *Marihuana: The Forbidden Medicine.* In an article in *High Times,* he argues that the huge amount of anecdotal evidence on medical cannabis should be considered as a validation of its effectiveness:

> Like everyone else who has been working over decades to ensure that marijuana, with all that it has to offer, is allowed to take its proper place in our lives, I have been heartened by the rapidly growing pace at which it is gaining understanding as a safe and versatile medicine. In addition to the relief it offers to so many patients with a large array of symptoms and syndromes (almost invariably at less cost, both in toxicity and money, than the conventional drugs it replaces), it is providing those patients, their caregivers, and the people who are close to them an opportunity to see for themselves how useful and unthreatening its use is. It has been a long and difficult sell, but I think it is now generally believed (except by the United States government) that herbal marijuana as a medicine is here to stay.
>
> The evidence which underpins this status as a medicine is, unlike that of almost all other modern medicines, anecdotal. Ever since the mid-1960s, new medicines have been officially

approved through large, carefully controlled double-blind studies, the same path that marijuana might have followed had it not been placed in Schedule I of the Controlled Substances Act of 1970, which has made it impossible to do the kind of studies demanded for approval by the Food and Drug Administration. Anecdotal evidence commands much less attention than it once did, yet it is the source of much of our knowledge of synthetic medicines as well as plant derivatives. Controlled experiments were not needed to recognize the therapeutic potential of chloral hydrate, barbiturates, aspirin, curare, insulin or penicillin. And there are many more recent examples of the value of anecdotal evidence. It was in this way that the use of propranolol for angina and hypertension, of diazepam for status epilepticus (a state of continuous seizure activity), and of imipramine for childhood enuresis (bed-wetting) was discovered, although these drugs were originally approved by regulators for other purposes.

Today, advice on the use of marijuana to treat a particular sign or symptom, whether provided or not by a physician, is based almost entirely on anecdotal evidence. For example, let's consider the case of a patient who has an established diagnosis of Crohn's disease but gets little or no relief from conventional medicines (or even occasional surgery) and suffers from severe cramps, diarrhea and loss of weight. His cannabis-savvy physician—one who is aware of compelling anecdotal literature suggesting that it is quite useful in this syndrome—would not hesitate to recommend to this patient that he try using marijuana. He might say, "Look, I can't be certain that this will help you, but there is now considerable experience that marijuana has been very useful in treating the symptoms of this disorder, and if you use it properly, it will not hurt you one bit; so I would suggest you give it a try, and if it works, great—and if it does not, it will not have harmed you."

If this advice is followed and it works for this patient, he will report back that, indeed, his use of the drug has eliminated the symptoms and he is now regaining his weight; or that it doesn't work for him but he is no better or worse off than he was before he had a trial of marijuana. Particularly in states which have accommodated the use of marijuana as a medicine, this kind of exchange is not uncommon. Because the use of cannabis as a medicine is so benign, relative to most of the conventional medicines it competes with, knowledgeable physicians are less hesitant to recommend a trial.

One of the problems of accepting a medicine—particularly one whose toxicity profile is lower than most over-the-counter medicines—on the basis of anecdotal evidence alone is that it runs the risk of being oversold. For example, it is presently being recommended for many types of pain, some of which are not responsive to its analgesic properties. Nonetheless, in this instance, a failed trial of marijuana is not a serious problem; and at the very least, both patient and physician learn that the least toxic analgesic available doesn't work for this patient with this type of pain. Unfortunately, this kind of trial is not always benign.[15]

While Dr. Grinspoon encourages us to consider anecdotal reports about the efficacy of medical marijuana, he also shares his very serious concern that some patients may put much *too much faith* in widespread anecdotal reports on the Internet and in books which claim that it cured cancer. I suggest that you read Dr. Grinspoon's article in its entirety on the High Times website. He ends the article with this guidance and admonition to cancer patients:

There is little doubt that cannabis now may play some non-curative roles in the treatment of this disease (or diseases) because it is often useful to cancer patients who suffer from nausea, anorexia, depression, anxiety, pain and insomnia. However, while there is growing evidence from animal studies that it may shrink tumor cells and cause other promising salutary effects in some cancers, there is no present evidence that it cures any of the many different types of cancer. I think the day will come when it or some cannabinoid derivatives will be demonstrated to have cancer-curative powers, but in the meantime, we must be very cautious about what we promise these patients.[16]

New, More Medicinal Strains of Cannabis

As I touched on in Chapter 1, most people think of medical cannabis as one specific medicine when, in reality, each strain of cannabis is, in some ways, a different medicine from every other strain. What do we mean by the word *strain* as it relates to medical cannabis? If you are a layperson in the world of botany like me, you may be more familiar with the word *variety* to distinguish plants of the same species from one another. Just think about all of the different varieties of tomatoes that are available, ranging from large, juicy heirloom tomatoes to small cherry tomatoes—with numerous sizes and shapes in-between. There are over 25,000 strains of tomatoes in the world; even though they are all tomatoes, there are many differences among them, including their nutritional content, size, color, taste, and texture. Nobody knows how many strains of cannabis exist today; however, one expert tells me over 1,000 strains have been named.

THC (tetrahydrocannabinol) and CBD (cannabidiol) are just two of the 80 to 100 cannabinoids found in the cannabis plant. One or the other or a combination of THC and CBD are prominent in most strains, often representing 50 percent or more of the total cannabinoids that are present, while the other 78 to 98 cannabinoids combined make up the rest of the total.

Each of the cannabinoids—even those that are present in minute amounts—has its own unique properties and potential healing benefits. Just as with other herbs that are used for medicinal purposes, it is the synergy—or "entourage effect"—of all of the active chemical compounds that Nature graced the plant with, working together, that create the healing effects. Because the ratios of cannabinoids and other chemicals vary in each strain, each strain is unique. To an extent, each strain of cannabis is a different medicine. As research continues and even more strains are bred, more patients will find illness- and condition-specific strains that ease symptoms and bring greater healing to a wider range of health challenges.

Cannabis experts are working to breed new strains for specific health issues, leading to even greater degrees of symptom relief and improved well-being for many patients. This is a total turnaround from the breeding practices of the illegal trade, which was driven by recreational users who wanted the increasingly bigger "highs" that came from larger ratios of THC. In fact, many of these recreational strains contained almost *no* CBD. And that's unfortunate since studies show that CBD has many healing properties.

Some media reports make it seem as if today's patients can easily obtain specific strains that have been proven to help with specific conditions. But, as of this writing, that's still rare. In most cases, patients are left on their own to determine the cannabis product or products that will work for them—and then obtaining them is not always easy. When I first became a medical cannabis patient, I learned this lesson quickly.

In my state, the doctor who gave me the "recommendation" that made it legal for me to obtain cannabis was not allowed to tell me what to buy or even where to go to obtain it. I had a piece of paper that said it was legal for me to buy medical marijuana but it was up to me to figure out what and where. It's hard to imagine this in the world of medicine; and even in the world of herbs there's not a good parallel. The closest analogy I could come up with is this: Let's say your doctor wrote you a prescription for an antibiotic. But, instead of writing down which of the 100-plus antibiotics she wanted you to take, she simply wrote "antibiotic" on the prescription, signed it, and sent you off to the pharmacy with it. The pharmacist would be flummoxed and, of course, unable to fill the prescription. That's basically what happens when patients are given the paperwork that allows them to purchase medical marijuana.

Medicinal cannabis strains are bred for their specific healing qualities and require quality control in the growing and manufacturing processes to ensure that they are of high quality, with no molds, pesticides, or other toxins or impurities. Since many patients have compromised immune systems, organic cannabis is preferable. In addition, treatment protocols for medical use of cannabis allow for non-intoxicating, smokeless, and topical forms and formulations.

Much of the cannabis that's available today, especially for recreational purposes, contains many times more THC than a few decades ago. CBD was, to a great extent, bred out of cannabis over the years by those in the illegal marijuana trade who were focused on providing high-THC content for customers. After all, most of them wanted the biggest high possible. Since the advent of medical cannabis in this modern era of the plant, efforts to breed higher-CBD content into some medical strains has been an ongoing challenge. It takes a long time, lots of patience, and a lot of know-how to breed new strains that have a specific chemical profile; therefore, while some medical cannabis growers and manufacturers are now focusing on high-CBD strains, the majority of the medical cannabis that has been available to date contains little to no CBD.

Another factor that must be considered in strain development is that just because more CBD is desirable, that does not mean THC is undesirable or should be bred out entirely. Depending on a patient's health condition and symptoms, different ratios of CBD and THC—and all of the additional chemicals that are natural to the plant—can make a big difference in the degree of its efficacy. It's also possible that two patients with the same diagnosis may find that different cannabis products—with different ratios of CBD, THC, and other chemicals—will be more effective for each of them. That being said, since CBD has been all but absent or in extremely low quantities until recently, the advent of new strains that are high in this healing chemical is advantageous to many.

The only difference between a high-CBD product that is "legal everywhere" and one that falls under medical marijuana laws is the amount of THC in it. The phrase "legal everywhere" is in quotes here because this is a gray area in many jurisdictions. It's possible that some high-CBD products that are legal today—or quasi-legal to the extent that governments are not stopping their sale—will be illegal in the future. Or, the tide could turn in a direction that I prefer with even more "legal everywhere" products that are high in quality and medically beneficial.

There are three basic types of high-CBD products currently available to patients:

1. High-CBD strains that are *so* low in THC that they are **considered to be legal nutritional supplements** and NOT medical marijuana in most jurisdictions.
2. High-CBD strains that also contain a fair amount of THC and are **considered to be medical marijuana**.
3. High-CBD strains that are **consumed in a raw form**, usually as cannabis juice or cannabis oil that has been cold processed. In most jurisdictions, these strains are **considered to be medical marijuana.** (See the

sections on Raw Cannabis below and also later in this book.)

In the first category above are high-CBD cannabis products that contain only a tiny amount of THC and are now legally sold in many jurisdictions as hemp foods and nutritional products. Because these strains have been bred to have extremely low quantities of THC), the chemical compound that causes psychoactivity or a "stoned feeling," and naturally high quantities of CBD, they are referred to as *hemp* in the U.S.—and referred to by some as "marijuana's sober cousin" since it is not possible to get high from them. (I'll share more specifics on CBD, THC, and the other cannabinoids in a later chapter.)

While the U.S. government has not established standards for the level of THC that is allowed in nutritional hemp products, as of this writing "trace" amounts are acceptable, even though a specific limit is not given. Canada and Europe do set limits; Canada's current law says that the THC level in a nutritional or industrial hemp plant must be under 0.3 percent of the total cannabinoids, while 1 percent is allowed in Europe.

New Product Trends

As new strains of cannabis are developed to address specific health conditions, there are two product trends that have become popular—cannabis oil and raw cannabis, both of which are covered in more detail later in this book. As an introduction, here's a brief overview:

Cannabis Oil

Earlier, I told you about *cannabis oil*, a concentrated cannabis product that is extremely potent. How does its potency compare with more traditional ways of taking cannabis, such as smoking a joint? One expert suggests that a patient who smokes marijuana joints would need to smoke hundreds per day to get the same benefits as one day's dosage of the more-potent cannabis oil. No one really knows *why* this type of oil is so much more potent than other forms of cannabis. Yes, it is concentrated, but so are other medical cannabis products.

One medical cannabis expert suggested to me that there may be some type of quantum physics transmutation going on in the extraction and processing of the oil that adds to its potency. That made me think about homeopathic remedies. While the process of making cannabis oil is totally different from the dilution and potentization process for homeopathic remedies, in both cases the result is a substance that's much more potent than it would be otherwise. We don't really know *why* this processing makes cannabis so potent, but I do know that many credit this oil, and products made from it, for their healing.

Cannabis oil can be made from any strain. Also, as you'll learn in Chapter 18, some cannabis oils are made with cold processing methods rather than heat. When manufactured with the proper methods, cold processing creates a cannabis oil that is non-psychoactive because it is technically still in its raw state. It is available in a syringe or small screw-top container. The type of syringe used for this purpose doesn't have a needle; just a tube with a cap on the end that is removed when you use it. Then, when you press on the syringe's plunger, the cannabis oil is pushed through it and out of the open end of the tube. The cap is then replaced until the next time you dispense oil from the syringe.

Cannabis oil can be taken on its own and it is also available in products such as capsules, lozenges, ointments, and suppositories. Until recently, most cannabis oil was very high in THC; however, as I mentioned earlier, new cannabis oil products that have been manufactured with cold-processing methods are now available. Since the cannabis is not actually heated in the processing, it is still in a raw state. That means it contains the precursor chemical THCa, which does not cause psychoactivity. These new raw products also contain high levels of CBD and also other cannabinoids such as CBG, which are more healing for some conditions.

Cannabis oil is also known by a host of other names. Because of his pioneering work with this type of oil, you'll notice that some of those names pay homage to Canadian farmer Rick Simpson: Rick Simpson Oil, Rick Simpson's *Hemp* Oil, RSO (for Rick Simpson Oil), RSHO (for Rick Simpson Hemp Oil), Hash Oil, or Honey Oil. For clarification, the use of the word *hemp* in the names of some of these oils is a bit confusing because, as I've said before, in the U.S. and some other parts of the world, *hemp* refers to strains of cannabis that are used only for nutritional and industrial products. However, in Canada, where Simpson is from, all types of cannabis are referred to as *hemp*, including those that are used for medicinal purposes.

At this point in time, without uniform standards for medical marijuana, the quality of any cannabis product depends on the professionalism and ethics of the manufacturer who is selling it. Some products that have no connection with Simpson use his name or the initials RSO or RSHO as a marketing tool. And sadly, many products, including some that erroneously imply a connection to Simpson, have been found to contain toxic metals, mold, and/or pesticides, which can be harmful to any patient. In this book, it is my goal to provide you with the information you need to be discerning in making these choices.

Raw Cannabis

Dr. William Courtney of Northern California is at the forefront of the raw cannabis movement, which I find promising because of the many stories of results with raw cannabis juice and other raw products. The biggest difference with raw cannabis products compared to all other forms of cannabis is that *psychoactivity* rarely occurs when cannabis is raw. The reason for this is the fact that raw cannabis contains little to no THC, the chemical that causes psychoactivity. Instead, raw cannabis contains THCa, the "acid" form of THC, which is a biosynthetic precursor to THC, as well as CBDa, the "acid" precursor to CBD. As with all cannabinoids, THCa and CBDa have unique healing benefits; however, the "acid" form of these chemicals may not be efficacious for all patients.

I'll go into more detail on raw cannabis and also discuss the rare cases in which it can cause psychoactivity in Chapter 19.

New Strains and Options that Cause NO Psychoactivity or LESS Psychoactivity

New cannabis product options are available with a low amount of THC (tetrahydrocannabinol). In most cases, they produce less psychoactivity OR no psychoactivity. Below is an overview of the types of products that fall in this category. However, please keep in mind that a low-THC product may not be efficacious for you. I'll explain more on all of this in later chapters.

1. **New High-CBD Strains of Cannabis**
   As we reviewed earlier in this chapter, new strains that are high in the chemical CBD (cannabidiol) are getting a lot of attention because of its numerous healing properties. High-CBD cannabis is now available in two sub-categories; the major difference between them is the amount of THC they contain—and that, in turn, relates to the level of psychoactivity they may cause. The sub-categories are:

A. *Nutritional Supplements* that Cause NO Psychoactivity

Some high-CBD strains contain such a small amount of THC—less than one percent in most cases—that they should not cause psychoactivity; these strains are generally referred to as "hemp" rather than marijuana or cannabis. They **do not** fall under medical marijuana laws in most jurisdictions and, therefore, are legally being sold as nutritional supplements. However, the legality of these products is a gray area right now, with some medical marijuana experts concerned that the U.S. government will crack down on them.

B. *Medical Cannabis Products* that Cause LESS Psychoactivity

Another category of newer high-CBD products contains enough THC to cause *some* psychoactivity, therefore they are legally considered to be marijuana. However, these strains have been bred to have a much higher amount of CBD, the chemical that has considerable healing benefits.

2. Raw Cannabis Products

Raw cannabis also fits in this category because, as discussed in the section above, when it's raw—and has not been exposed to heat—cannabis almost never causes psychoactivity. (See Chapter 19 for the rare exceptions to this.)

Chapter 4

Why the Chemistry of Marijuana Proves That It's a Unique Superherb

When I first landed in the medical marijuana world, the experts I relied upon were a friend of a friend and the guy who is called the "budtender" at the nearby marijuana collective. I remember the excitement of both of them as they told me about the human body's *endocannabinoid system*, which is so named because it is a "match" for the cannabinoids in cannabis. To them, it meant that something amazing and unique was going on because, as they both explained, the main chemical compounds in cannabis are *the same* as the cannabinoid receptors in the bodies of all mammals, including us humans. But it didn't make much sense to me because I couldn't understand why a "system" in the body was named for a plant. As I learned more, I finally started to understand *why* the discovery of endocannabinoids was considered to be a huge breakthrough.

The Discovery That Proves Why Cannabis Is So Healing

As I mentioned in Chapter 1, these compounds in the human body—called endocannabinoids—were not identified until the 1990s, when pioneering researchers were able to connect the dots. They discovered for the first time that chemical compounds in cannabis, which are called cannabinoids, are a match for receptors in our own cells. As a result, because the cannabinoids in marijuana actually match these receptors in the body, the scientists honored the herb by naming the body's own newly-discovered internal version after it. They added the prefix "endo," which means "in, within, inside," to the word "cannabinoid" to create the word "endocannabinoid."

Scientists discovered that the body's endocannabinoid system is involved in a variety of physiological processes including appetite, pain sensation, and memory. In fact, they now view the endocannabinoid system as the largest neurotransmitter system in the body. Here's an excerpt from an article by Allan Badiner that does a great job of explaining the science of endocannabinoids:

> The science of endocannabinoid medicine has progressed to a dizzying degree in the past few years. There is wider awareness that the "endocannabinoid system" is the largest neurotransmitter system in the human body, regulating relaxation, eating, sleeping, memory, and, as noted by the Italian scientist Vincenzo Di Marzo, even our immune system.
>
> Cannabinoids promote homeostasis, the maintenance of a stable internal environment despite external fluctuations, at every level of biological life, from the sub-cellular, to the organism. For example, endocannabinoids are now understood as the source of the runner's high. The endocannabinoids naturally found in human breast milk, which are vital for proper human development, have virtually identical effects as cannabinoids found in the cannabis plant...
>
> Universally accepted following its discovery in 1995, the endocannabinoid system asserts its power to heal and balance the other systems of the body by turning on or off the expression of genes. Cannabinoids hold the key that unlocks

receptor sites throughout the brain and immune system triggering potent healing and pain-killing effects.[17]

And that's what my two new friends were so excited about; the endocannabinoid system is a link between this specific plant and our health. In Chapter 1, we looked at the way receptor sites on the surface of cells can lock onto certain molecules when they come along, basically working like locks and keys. This same type of mechanism is at play when the cannabinoids in cannabis match the receptors in the body's endocannabinoid system like a "lock and key." I like the way this cellular interaction is explained on the website http://canna-centers.com:

> The cannabinoids interact with the receptors, much like a lock and key. The receptor is the lock and the cannabinoid molecule is the key. When the cannabinoid "key" attaches to the receptor "lock" (located on a cell wall), a reaction is triggered resulting in an effect on the brain and body. For instance, the area of the brain that controls memories is called the amygdala. When cannabinoids bind to the receptors on the cells of the amygdala, memory is affected. For those that suffer from past traumatic events who relive horrible memories (such as those with Post Traumatic Stress Disorder), the triggering of the cannabinoid receptor appears to change the brain function and memories are minimized.[18]

Let's focus on the 75 trillion cells in your body for a moment. The cell is the biological unit of any living organism. You have skin cells, heart cells, hair cells, cornea cells—every part of your body contains cells that are dedicated to their own specific function. Cells are referred to as the building blocks of life; the fact is, your body lives and dies on a cellular level. Every moment of every day your cells are at work—and each one of those 75 trillion cells is like a little factory, with components that work synergistically with other cells to perform numerous functions. When your cells are healthy, they function properly and the body is constantly in the process of healing itself. In fact, *this very second*, millions of cells in your body that have been damaged by oxidative stress, bacteria, viruses, and free radical damage will die and, automatically, they will be replaced by new cells as they go through their normal "repair or replace" function.

Researchers can now see deep into the cells and are working to map all of their intricate processes. In his book, *The Science of Healing Revealed: New Insights into Redox Signaling*, atomic and medical physicist Dr. Gary Samuelson explains just how intricate these processes are. He asks us to look at life from the cell's point-of-view:

> If we were to dive down inside the cell … we would see a bustling metropolis of thousands of different types of molecular actors floating around in the salt water, full of activity, extending for hundreds of yards in all directions; proteins being manufactured and folded, delivery systems of microtubules taxiing these proteins around to where they need to go, receptors receiving and transferring messages from inside and outside the cell and factory-like organelles, hubs where the most complex manufacturing takes place. … Within this thriving buzz of activity is found the mystery of human cellular life.[19]

When we give our bodies cannabis medicine, the matching receptors in our cells greet it in a synergistic way. The cannabis assists the entire system in effectively handling biological functions— as well as dealing with any challenges to those functions. The endocannabinoid system in the body modulates or balances every human physiological system, including regulating immunity, inflammation, neurotoxicity, blood pressure, appetite, gastro-intestinal function, and intraocular pressure.

In their book, *Cannabis Chemotherapy: The Science of Treating and Preventing Cancer with Concentrated Marijuana Medicine,* researcher David Hoye and his coauthors explain the role of the human endocannabinoid system in dealing with cancerous cells:

> The human endocannabinoid system ... has been found to play a major part in controlling the natural process that makes healthy cells die off when they are supposed to, instead of continuing to grow into cancerous tumors. In addition, a healthy and functioning endocannabinoid system prevents malignant cells from growing special blood vessels to feed tumor growth, thereby starving it to death instead of feeding it.
>
> It is surmised that a healthy, well-regulated endo-cannabinoid system keeps the ever-opportunistic cancer cells from developing and growing. When this system slows down or turns off, cancer cells are given a favorable environment for their growth and the disease develops. **The plant-derived cannabinoids in marijuana activate the same receptors as do the internally-produced endo-cannabinoids.** [Emphasis mine] Therefore, when the internal system lets down its defense, a similar effect on the cannabinoid receptors can be created through use of plant-derived cannabinoids. This is how cannabis medicine activates and stimulates the body's own cancer-fighting mechanisms.
>
> In addition to stimulating the body's own cancer-fighting systems, **cannabinoids have been shown to kill malignant cancer cells they contact, while sparing or, according to some studies, actually strengthening the normal healthy cells adjacent to the cancerous**

growth. [Emphasis mine] It is remarkable how many different ways the active elements in marijuana fight against cancer, even using different mechanisms to counteract different forms of the disease.[20]

Another function of the endocannabinoid system is its role as a set of *signaling molecules* in the central and peripheral nervous system. The endocannabinoid system is one of various classes or types of signaling molecules through which cells communicate with each other. These signaling molecules are messengers that transmit information from one to another—in some cases over long distances and, in other cases, between cells that are right next door to each other. They direct thousands of chemical reactions that take place inside and outside each cell every second and, as they do so, they carry out instructions on when and how the chemical reactions are to take place. As some cells become diseased or damaged, these signaling molecules have a critical role to play in the repair process. They signal the cell's defenses to take action. If the cell cannot fix itself, the signaling molecules enable the destruction of the unhealthy cell and it is then replaced by a new healthy cell. At least, that is what happens when the cells are working properly.

As we deal with toxins in our food, air, water, and environment; toxic thinking from limited or negative beliefs; and the process of aging, cells can become damaged or inefficient and stop operating at full power. These impaired cells begin duplicating themselves rather than purposely destroying themselves as they were instructed. When that happens, the body is stuck with the damaged or lazy cells instead of the new healthy cells that it requires for optimum health. As a result, our immune system weakens, causing illness and disease to creep in and, sometimes, stay with us. We then develop chronic pain, symptoms of old age, slowed ability to heal, and decay. In some cases, this malfunction of signaling causes uncontrolled growth of the cells. The body is supposed to eliminate these runaway cells—but when conditions don't trigger the repair or replace mechanism to eliminate and replace them with new, healthy cells, the runaway cells continue to multiply. In fact, many people have pockets of infection in their bodies that they aren't even aware of. Over time, if the immune system is unable to eliminate the infection, it can wreak havoc on the body's health.

Let's review some definitions:

- *Cannabinoids* are chemical compounds in the cannabis plant that bind to and activate receptors in our own cells.
- *Endocannabinoids* are cannabinoid substances our bodies naturally make, which are activated by the chemicals in the cannabis plant.

When the discovery of the body's endocannabinoid system was made, scientists were clearly aware of the humor and the irony of the situation, given this particular herb's complex, confusing, and checkered history. As I mentioned earlier, a 2004 article in *Scientific American* didn't shy away from the obvious; it was titled "The Brain's Own Marijuana." The article was summarized this way: "Research into natural chemicals that mimic marijuana's effects in the brain could help to explain—and suggest treatments for—pain, anxiety, eating disorders, phobias and other conditions."[21]

The *Scientific American* article explained:

> **Everyone grows a form of the drug, regardless of their political leanings or recreational proclivities. That is because the brain makes its own marijuana, natural compounds called endocannabinoids (after the plant's formal name, Cannabis sativa).** [Emphasis mine]
>
> The study of endocannabinoids in recent years has led to exciting discoveries. By examining these substances, researchers have exposed an entirely new signaling system in

the brain: a way that nerve cells communicate that no one anticipated even 15 years ago. Fully understanding this signaling system could have far-reaching implications. The details appear to hold a key to devising treatments for anxiety, pain, nausea, obesity, brain injury and many other medical problems.[22]

The article also tells us that some of the body's endocannabinoids are located "in parts of the brain associated with complex motor behavior, cognition, learning, and memory."[23]

When these signaling agents are not in proper number and balance, the body begins to deteriorate. That deterioration can come through illness, injury, or simply the process of aging. As we age, even the healthiest body produces fewer and fewer signaling molecules, which are diminished by about ten percent per decade. That's why a five-year-old who scrapes her knee heals so much faster than a 50-year-old with the same type of injury. In fact, scientists now believe that the decrease in signaling molecules is the actual mechanism that causes our body to age.

But Wait, There's More—One of the Endocannabinoids in Your Body Causes Bliss!

In 1992, scientists at Hebrew University in Israel discovered that one of the endocannabinoids in the human brain and nervous system is, at least in part, responsible for the blissful or pleasurable feelings that you experience. They named it by taking the Sanskrit word *ananda*, which means *bliss*, and adding "amide" to the end, calling it *anandamide*.

While anandamide is just one of the endocannabinoids in your body, to date it's one of the most fascinating to researchers. That's because the pharmacologic properties of anandamide are also in THC, the chemical compound in cannabis that causes psychoactivity. That means when we ingest THC, anandamide is activated in the body, primarily in the brain and the immune system.

In a later chapter, I'll get into more details about THC and some of the other cannabinoids; right now, let's go a bit deeper in our exploration of the "bliss" chemical, anandamide with this excerpt from an article written by Helga George:

> Anandamide is synthesized when needed. It is not stored in cells. The compound does not last long and is quickly degraded by a number of enzymes. In particular, it is degraded by fatty acid amide hydrolase, which releases fatty acid breakdown products into the cell.
>
> It was thought that anandamide was released from cellular membranes and diffused short distances to its active site. This would be unlike traditional hormones that travel long distances in the body. There is some evidence suggesting that this molecule might be carried within cells in structures composed of fatty molecules....
>
> The discovery of anandamide was a significant finding and unleashed a whole field of study on similar compounds. This compound is derived from lipids — in particular, a fatty acid called arachidonic acid. There is some evidence that the amount of arachidonic acid in the diet can affect the amount of anandamide in the body.[24]

While its role in assisting us with motivation and pleasure led to the naming of anandamide, studies have also found that it plays a role in the regulation of eating, provides analgesic effects that are induced by exercise, and inhibits proliferation of breast cancer cells. An article on the website General Chemistry Online explains more on the important roles anandamide plays in our health and well-being:

Anandamide is synthesized enzymatically in areas of the brain that are important in memory and higher thought processes, and in areas that control movement. That implies that anandamide's function is not just to produce bliss. ...

Connections between nerve cells are associated with learning and memory. Nerve cells can make new connections and break old ones. Repeated use of a connection makes it grow stronger; lack of use can cause the connection to be lost. Some biochemical evidence suggests that anandamide plays a role in the making and breaking of short term neural connections [Derkinderen, 1996].[25]

Another fascinating function of anandamide is its role in female reproduction by assisting in the implantation of the early stage fetal cells into the uterus. This fascinating aspect of one of anandamide's specific functions is discussed in the same online article:

Outside the brain, anandamide acts as a chemical messenger between the embryo and uterus during implantation of the embryo in the uterine wall. As such, it's one of the first communications that occurs between mother and child.

The highest concentrations of anandamide in the body were not in the brain, but in the uterus just before embryo implantation (at least, in the animal studies done so far) [KUMC, 1996]. The concentration of anandamide changes as the uterus becomes more receptive to embryo implantation. The researchers were able to locate a definite target for the uterus' anandamide signal: mouse embryos contain more anandamide receptors than any tissue known, including the brain.[26]

Another interesting aspect of anandamide is the way it functions with stress. People with chronic stress, including post-traumatic stress disorder (PTSD), have *less* anandamide concentrated in their bodies.

As I said earlier, anandamide is perhaps the most fascinating endocannabinoid in the body; however, it's just one endocannabinoid. As science continues to study the ways in which our bodies and cannabis work together synergistically, other endocannabinoids or other types of chemicals may be found to have equally fascinating properties and functions.

Augmenting and Activating the Endocannabinoid System with Cannabis

Can healthy people benefit from cannabis too? Some experts believe that even the most healthy among us would benefit from taking a small amount of cannabis daily along with our other nutritional supplements. If your doctor is on the leading edge of health and nutrition, it's possible that one day she will recommend that you take a low-dose cannabis product on a daily basis to activate your endocannabinoid system. Use of a low-dose cannabis product, such as a tonic or a raw whole plant cannabis tablet in the range of 5 to 10 milligrams may one day be as standard as taking a multi-vitamin supplement is today for many people.

Interesting research conducted in Israel has shown that the protective effects of cannabis may also be helpful for brain health. Professor Yosef Sarne of Tel Aviv University found that patients suffering from brain injuries experienced a significant reduction in long-term brain damage when they were given cannabis as part of their treatment. To me, a fascinating aspect of this research is that the beneficial results were about the same for patients whether they were taking cannabis *before* or *after* their injury. That information definitely points to the health-giving benefits of taking cannabis on a regular basis.[27]

Chapter 5

Why the Healing Synergy of Nature's Medicines Is Important

Before we focus on the specific chemical compounds in cannabis, it's helpful to look at the reasons why many people prefer herbs and other natural medicines to pharmaceutical drugs, finding them to be safer, less expensive and, often, more effective. According to archeologists, medicinal herbs have been used to heal and to promote wellness as far back as human history has been recorded.

Nature's Medicines Bring Healing—And Other Benefits Too

While each herb has its own unique chemical makeup, many have been found to boost the immune system, increase vitality, and increase resistance to infections. Food herbs, including common herbs such as parsley and basil, add healthy nutrients and other beneficial chemical compounds to our diets and can be used in just about any quantity. However, medicinal herbs, such as valerian, kava kava, Echinacea, goldenseal, St. John's wort, calendula, and many more, have been known to have much greater healing potential than food herbs—and they should be respected as the medicines they are. Even a seemingly benign herb like valerian, which many people routinely take, can cause liver damage if taken in excess over a period of time.

When a person's health is out of sync to a degree that it is impeding her lifestyle, it's common for us to view the symptoms as evidence of a disease or injury. However, the cells of your body don't think of the symptoms as the flu or cancer or sprained ankle. The cells simply spring into action and do whatever they can to deal with the symptoms and heal the condition. To the best of its ability, the innate wisdom of your body begins the process of healing simultaneously with the onset of the symptom or injury.

Over the last couple of decades, much has changed in the world of holistic health as more and more people want natural, holistic and organic products that their bodies respond to positively. They want products that don't have the negative side effects that are pervasive with most pharmaceutical drugs, some of which are debilitating and addictive. The good news is that with herbs and other natural treatments, the side effects, if any, are almost always beneficial *as long as they are used in appropriate ways and with appropriate dosages.* But that's not the case with pharmaceutical drugs. Each year huge numbers of people are prescribed pharmaceutical painkillers, sleeping pills, and other drugs that can be dangerous and addictive. Just read the labels and the ads.

In most cases, when a patient takes the appropriate dosage of a strain of cannabis that is efficacious for them, they experience a degree of symptom relief along with the added benefit of the overall healing qualities of the herb. In contrast, when we take pharmaceutical drugs, the drug sometimes becomes less effective as the body becomes tolerant to it. And, should one stop taking the drug, the potential withdrawal symptoms may be difficult to handle, especially if the body is still in a weakened state due to illness. With cannabis, a patient may want to take more to increase the benefits as tolerance develops but, other than the possibility of having to deal with a psychoactive high or stoned feeling if you are taking cannabis that contains THC, there are few potentially negative side effects.

When I was dependent on pharmaceutical drugs, I needed to take more and more to get the same benefits. I found myself getting up in the middle of the night to take additional pills. Even though I wasn't supposed to take more than the prescribed dose, that was the only way

I could get back to sleep and get enough sleep to function the next day. But I don't find the benefits of cannabis to be dosage-dependent. I have switched from a very high dose one night to a much lower dose the next and achieved the same benefits. I have even skipped a few nights on cannabis because I simply forgot to take it. I recall lying in bed, waiting for the wave of relaxation that it gives me, and then realizing that I hadn't taken it. I could have gotten up but I was close to sleep and elected not to do so. I didn't sleep as well on those nights when I didn't take the cannabis—and sometimes it took quite a while to get to sleep—but I did sleep. That was in strong contrast to being on the pharmaceutical drugs that, over time, my body seemed to *require* in order to sleep.

Understanding the Differences Between Herbal Medicine and Pharmaceuticals

An understanding of the differences between herbal medicine and pharmaceuticals is helpful here. One of the leading voices in holistic health is Harvard trained medical doctor and author Dr. Andrew Weil, who also has a degree in botany and therefore an understanding of the natural world that's rooted in science. It's interesting to note that up until the early to mid-1800s, all doctors studied botany because almost all medicines were made from plants. That's where doctors got their medicines—from Nature. Today, some pharmaceutical drugs are still made from compounds of herbs while others are synthetic versions of those compounds.

In his book, *Health and Healing*, Dr. Weil explains why it is so important that we value *all* of the chemical compounds in a medicinal plant, rather than determining that some compounds are more important than others. He tells us that when one or more active components are extracted out of an herb, its potential for healing is diminished because it is no longer in the state that Nature provided. Dr. Weil says:

> I am afraid the choices of medical scientists in modifying natural drugs have also mostly been foolish, because they have valued increased potency and pharmacological power and rapid action over safety and overall quality of effect. Some of their creations have been true blessings, many more are mixed blessings, and **some have been curses to humanity**. [Emphasis mine][28]

I suspect that Dr. Weil's reference to pharmaceutical drugs that were "curses to humanity" is about drugs that were touted as breakthroughs, but then, after inflicting great harm to patients—sometimes even causing deaths—were pulled from the market.

The term *entourage effect* has been used to explain why all of the chemicals in cannabis are considered important—and why a synthetic version of the plant that includes some, but not all, of its chemical compounds is often found to be less efficacious. A story that Dr. Weil shares in *Health and Healing* explains why the entourage effect is considered important. Dr. Weil says he was very confused when the heart medication digitalis was taught in his medical school pharmacology class. Digitalis is a potent heart medication which is given in minute doses. It is such a potent drug that it must be precisely dosed for each patient and requires close medical supervision for safe use. The pharmaceutical text explained that there were three successive stages that were indicators of overdosing or drug toxicity. By carefully monitoring a patient and catching any problems at the early stages, the doctor could alter the dosage and keep the patient safe. The first indicator that the dosage was too high was gastrointestinal symptoms, usually nausea and vomiting. The second indicator was more serious and showed up as benign or atrial arrhythmias of the heart, which means that the upper chambers of the heart beat in abnormal rhythms. And the third stage, which can be fatal in minutes, is ventricular arrhythmia, in which the main or lower chambers of the heart beat irregularly.

Even though these three successive stages were taught in the medical textbooks, pharmacological manuals, and classes, Dr. Weil and his fellow students got conflicting information from their medical school instructors, all of whom said that the first stage—nausea and vomiting—*never* occurs. Instead, the first indicator that patients were experiencing an overdose or toxicity to the drug was the much more serious arrhythmia of the heart, which is stage two. Then, if they weren't treated in a timely fashion, they could quickly go into the life-threatening stage three. That didn't make any sense. Dr. Weil asked why there is a stage one if it never happens? But no one had the answer. They taught it this way *because they were taught it this way.* And, even though the information was clearly not accurate, apparently no one had the audacity to change the wording in the textbook.

Some years after medical school, as Dr. Weil was talking with an older doctor, they discussed their common belief that plant forms of drugs are relatively safe. Then, surprisingly, the older doctor provided the answer to the riddle of why students were taught about the phantom "stage one" indicator of a digitalis overdose. It seems the original form of digitalis was the herb foxglove. When foxglove was given to heart patients in its natural form, the dosage could be easily monitored because of a chemical compound in the plant that caused them to get sick to the stomach if they were taking too much. That's where the nausea and vomiting came into the picture. But when digitalis, the main chemical compound in foxglove, was extracted and isolated and sold as a pharmaceutical drug, the chemical compounds in the plant that could cause the minor stomach upset were no longer present. So, unlike their predecessors who dispensed the herb itself, modern doctors who prescribe the pharmacological version, digitalis, do not have the advantage of the stage one "early warning" symptom. Rather, the first indication that a patient might be overdosing is much more serious and even potentially life-threatening.

Back in the day when the foxglove plant was given to patients in its natural form, the synergistic compounds in the plant worked together and the patient's own body would signal any dosing adjustments that were needed by causing nausea and vomiting. Dr. Weil explains:

> In their enthusiasm at isolating the active principles of drug plants, researchers of the last century made a serious mistake. They came to believe that all of a plant's desirable properties could be accounted for by a single compound, that it would always be better to conduct research and treat disease with the purified compound than with the whole plant. In this belief, they forgot the plants once they had the active principles out of them, called the other principles "inactive," and advanced the notion that prescribing refined white powders was more scientific and up-to-date than using crude green plants....
>
> The erroneous idea that plants and isolated active principles are equivalent has become the dogma in pharmacology and medicine today. Drug plants are always complex mixtures of chemicals, all of which contribute to the effect of the whole. In general, isolated and refined drugs are

much more toxic than their botanical sources. They also tend to produce effects of more rapid onset, greater intensity and shorter duration. Sometimes they fail to reproduce desirable actions of plants they come from, and sometimes they lack natural safeguards present in those plants. Our problems stem directly from the decision of scientific medicine to value the refined white powder over the green plant.

The possibility that secondary compounds of medicinal plants may be valuable in their own right or may modify the effects of dominant compounds in good ways seems unremarkable to me. Nevertheless, I find I have to explain it to allopathic physicians and pharmacologists with great patience. I notice that I make many of these people uneasy when I impute any "wisdom" to nature. They seem to resent the suggestion that natural substances may be better than manmade ones. All that I can say is that, empirically, I have found such a difference, at least in the case of medicinal plants versus isolated drugs. Whenever I have had a chance to observe or experience firsthand treatment with a plant and treatment with a refined derivative of the plant, I have found the latter to be more dangerous and sometimes less useful.[29]

A Primer on the Drug-Creation Process

Rather than focus on the natural plant, which cannot be patented and therefore has limited income potential, pharmaceutical drug companies do considerable research to find the molecular basis of a disease. Then they continue to research until they come up with a compound that will alter the patient's chemistry and block the receptors the body uses that causes the problem. For example, let's say a person has high blood pressure. That patient's blood pressure is high because a specific receptor in the body has been activated. The pharmaceutical option is to give the person a drug that will block that receptor so the blood pressure cannot go too high. But the pharmaceutical drug doesn't heal the cause of the high blood pressure. Instead of assisting the body to come back into balance, the drug masks the symptom, causing even more of a disturbance. And that can lead to more health challenges, not the healing that we so desperately want. It's understandable that doctors prefer medicines that are uniform in potency so they can accurately dose a patient and, hopefully, get specific effects each time they prescribe the medication. But some consider this to be a "magic bullet" approach and believe that it is generally not the most effective.

Another of my favorite holistic doctors is Dr. Joseph Mercola, who publishes an e-newsletter through his website, http://www.Mercola.com, which is filled with extremely well-researched articles. Dr. Mercola wrote an excellent review of a documentary called *Pill Poppers*, part of which I'm sharing below. Brace yourself; although this excerpt is a bit lengthy, it's only part of his review of this film, which provides an enlightened look at *how* many pharmaceutical drugs are developed. I urge you to read it carefully as it provides an excellent primer on the "drug-creation" process. I also highly suggest that you follow the link in my endnote and read the entire review on Dr. Mercola's website.

> Despite what the media preaches to you, your body has no intrinsic need for drugs. Over the course of a lifetime, the average person may be prescribed 14,000 pills (this doesn't even include over-the-counter meds), and by the time you reach your 70s you could be taking five or more pills every day, according to *Pill Poppers*, a documentary.
>
> The featured film asks a poignant question that anyone taking medications should also, which is, are these pills really beneficial, or are they doing more harm than good? ...

Pill Poppers takes you on a journey through some of the most popular drugs in the world, from the ADHD drug Ritalin to drugs for erectile dysfunction, depression, pain and contraception.

It starts out by taking you into a lab at GlaxoSmithKline (GSK), where 2 million chemical compounds are kept in a vault. Scientists know little about their effects; each could be lethal or lifesaving.

Through a process that could be described as finding a needle in a haystack, scientists methodically introduce a known disease molecule to each of the 2 million substances, one at a time, and assess whether anything happens.

If "something" happens, further tests are then conducted to find out what and why. Literally hundreds of millions of such tests are conducted, and it takes about $1 billion and an estimated 15 years of work to reach the ultimate goal: a licensed drug.

Despite what most are led to believe, just because the drug makes it through the regulatory process it's no guarantee of safety. Typically, more information is learned about a drug *after* it's been released to the market than before, because only then does it get the widespread exposure that clinical trials cannot simulate.

It's usually after millions of people have already started taking a drug that severe, sometimes deadly, side effects are observed, but unfortunately for some, it will be realized too late. As stated in the documentary: "Drugs are not designed but discovered, and we only find out what they really do to us when we take them."

Patrick Vallance, the head of drug discovery at GSK, even said, "In many ways you learn as much about your medicine after it's launched as you knew before." (Of course, GSK has also pleaded guilty to felony charges for knowingly manufacturing and selling adulterated drugs, a practice that adds even more of a "learning curve" when drugs are released...)

The Effects of Many Medications Are Discovered by Mistake

Many people assume that the medications they're taking are exerting carefully designed effects on specific biological pathways in their bodies. In reality, these effects were not designed but rather observed—often simply as a matter of sheer dumb luck—and the medication was then "discovered." The erectile dysfunction drug Viagra, for instance, was originally developed to treat angina. That it led to increased erections was simply a surprise.

The ADHD drug Ritalin was also discovered by accident, as it was originally designed to treat adults with depression. We're only now beginning to understand how this drug works, and what its long-term side effects entail, yet now it's already morphing into a drug with another purpose as a "study drug" for people without ADHD. And this is only a short list.

... Often, drugmakers and scientists are "surprised" to learn that their new blockbuster drug leads to unknown (or undisclosed) side effects, altering and disrupting far more functions in your body than was first realized. Viagra, for instance, can cause blue-green color blindness. And a commonly used class of diabetes drugs is now being investigated for causing pre-cancerous changes, with the antibiotic Zithromax (Z-Pak), may trigger lethal heart arrhythmias.

The truth is, no drug is side effect-free—a fact that many loyal pill takers are not aware of. These side effects are then often treated with ... even more drugs, perpetuating a vicious cycle. Even GSK's Vallance stated in the film: "When you make a medicine you're trying to disrupt a fundamental biological process. That's a pretty profound change, you can't do that without producing some unwanted effects—so then the question is, what risks are you prepared to take for what benefit?"

Creating Diseases to Fit the Treatments

Drug companies are masters at disease mongering—inventing non-existent diseases and exaggerating minor ones, with the end result making you rush to your doctor to request their drug solutions. It also misleads people into thinking drugs are the only option for every ill. Viagra is a perfect example, as it was originally intended only for men with actual erectile dysfunction. Many men have an occasional problem in this area, and that is normal, but Viagra is marketed in a way that makes it appear as though it's not.

Another blatant example of creating a market for a disease where none existed before is low female sex drive, or female sexual dysfunction, for which drug makers are actively seeking a "cure." One more example? In order to market its antidepressant Paxil, GSK hired a PR firm to create a public awareness campaign about an "under-diagnosed" disease.

The disease? Social anxiety disorder ... previously known as shyness. You may have seen this campaign firsthand a couple of years back; ads stating "Imagine being allergic to people" were distributed widely, celebrities gave interviews to the press and psychiatrists gave lectures on this new disease in the top 25 media markets. As a result, mentions of social anxiety in the press rose from about 50 to over 1 billion in just two years ... social anxiety disorder became the "third most common mental illness" in the US ... and Paxil skyrocketed to the top of the charts as one of the most profitable and most prescribed drugs in the US.

The Drug Industry is Now Trying to Treat Not Just Diseases but Risk Factors

The drug market is saturated with drugs to treat existing diseases and many drug firms are now trying to create markets for new drugs via disease-mongering. But another way to drum up business, which the industry is fully embracing, is using drugs to treat diseases you don't even have ....

If you have a "risk" of heart disease, for instance, which could apply to anyone aged 50 or over, you should be taking a statin, according to some "experts." Typically, statins are reserved for people considered to be at high risk of heart attack or stroke, usually (incorrectly) defined as someone with "high" cholesterol. The current value of the cholesterol-lowering drug industry is estimated at around $30 billion a year—but the pharmaceutical industry is still salivating at the thought of how big that number could get if statins could be prescribed to even more people. Alas, researchers came out with a study stating that even people at low risk of heart problems should take statins!

So even if you're healthy, you still need to be popping pills to preserve your health, according to the drug industry. Millions of others take drugs for reasons outside of health, such as contraception, or rely on them for functions for which there are far better solutions, such as weight loss, sleep or, in the case of using ADHA drugs for studying, increased focus or energy. Yet, disease is not the result of drug deficiency, nor will good health ever be the sole result of taking prescription drugs.[30]

Cannabis Medicines That Contain Isolated or Synthetic Chemicals

For many years, pharmaceutical companies have been working to create new drugs based on the specific chemical compounds that Nature endowed in cannabis and other herbs. They want to patent the chemicals they believe to be the most efficacious so they can control the marketplace. But why use their model at all? Why take a product that contains isolated or synthetic versions of THC or other cannabinoids if you can choose a cornucopia of Nature's bounty and wisdom by using a product that contains all of the beneficial chemicals in the plant? (THC and other cannabinoids are covered in depth in Chapter 7.)

Clearly, there are many good reasons for using all of the synergistic elements rather than singling out one or more compounds. In some parts of the world, holistic and natural approaches are still revered by many. For example, in China natural herbal drugs have traditionally been considered superior to pharmaceutical drugs because they focus on strengthening the body's defenses and internal resistance rather than attempting to cure a specific disease.

Another way that some medical cannabis experts are manipulating the chemical components of cannabis is by developing new strains that have no THC at all. By removing the THC, they are removing the psychoactive component that is troublesome for many people. But, unfortunately, they are also removing the healing benefits that THC gives to patients.

Keeping an open mind, it's certainly possible that cannabis with absolutely no THC would have fabulous healing properties, but most of the experts that I trust believe that all of Nature's ingredients are important—and I just can't see ditching the THC. Luckily, it doesn't have to be an "either/or" situation; newer strains of cannabis are being bred that have such a low level of THC that it causes little or no psychoactivity, but doesn't ditch the THC altogether.

Even though cannabis has been used throughout history for healing, today's medical cannabis experts have no idea what the chemical profiles were for strains that healers and doctors used in the past. It is entirely possible that many of those strains were very low in THC and very high in CBD, similar to the new medicinal strains that are being bred today. That's the exact opposite of the balance of these two chemicals in most, if not all, of the cannabis that's been available through illegal channels. But we don't want to get rid of the THC altogether because there's a reason Nature included it.

As I referenced earlier, the other new trend in the world of cannabis medicine is to use a raw form, which provides the benefits of THC without the accompanying psychoactivity, except in very rare cases. That's because, in its totally fresh, raw form, cannabis does not contain THC. Instead, it contains THCa, the biosynthetic precursor of THC, which has anti-inflammatory and neuroprotective effects. (The "a" at the end of THCa stands for "acid.") THCa does NOT cause psychoactivity; however, when cannabis is dried or heated for a period of time or burned or vaporized, the THCa converts to regular THC. If THCa is not heated, it is still THCa. Whether you choose raw cannabis juice or another form of raw cannabis, raw is a great way to go, especially if the healing qualities that are attributed specifically to THCa are preferable for you and/or you would like to take a non-psychoactive type of cannabis. (See Chapter 19 for the rare cases in which THCa can cause some degree of psychoactivity.)

Of course, herbal supplements are generally fairly inexpensive, especially when compared to many pharmaceutical drugs. I recently heard a new report on the extremely high cost of pharmaceutical cancer drugs. Even those who have good health insurance often find that their share of the cost is prohibitive, making the drugs out-of-reach for many. And the possible negative side effects that they bring with them can be equally distressing.

Iatrogenic Illnesses: The Rise in Health Challenges Caused by Drugs, Medical Treatments, and Procedures

We expect doctors to help us maintain well-being and to heal us when we're ill. However, some health challenges are iatrogenic in origin, which means they are *caused* by a drug, a medical treatment, or a diagnostic procedure that was prescribed or performed by a doctor or surgeon. The number of patients being diagnosed with iatrogenic conditions has been on the rise in recent decades, not on a decline. On this subject, Dr. Weil says:

> Adverse drug reactions account for the lion's share of iatrogenic illness so common that any dedicated patient is sure to experience one sooner or later. They can be as mild as nausea, hives, and drowsiness or as serious as permanent damage to organs and death. In addition to the adverse effects and interactions between drugs, other causes of iatrogenic illness are medication errors such as the wrong prescription or illegible handwriting causing the wrong drug or the wrong potency or dosage to be prescribed; over-use of drugs, such as antibiotic resistance; unnecessary surgery; negligence; and hospital-acquired infections.[31]

On a CNN special, Dr. Sanjay Gupta gave some frightening statistics about the problem that prescription drugs have become in the last few decades, including the fact that prescription drugs have replaced car crashes as the number one reason for accidental deaths in the U.S.[32]

In the report, Dr. Gupta went on to say that 75 percent of these accidental drug-caused deaths were caused by one category of drugs—and that category is painkillers.[33] In fact, it's shocking to learn that the U.S., which has just 5 percent of the world's population, consumes 80 percent of the painkillers that are prescribed around the world.

Another fascinating study focused on accidental deaths that were caused by patients who overdosed on painkillers, and to what extent those statistics differed in states where medical marijuana was legal. The researchers reviewed death certificate data in all 50 states in the U.S. for the period between 1999 and 2010 to determine how many people died as a result of prescription painkiller overdoses. Then, when they looked at the statistics from the 13 states where medical marijuana was legal during that timeframe, they determined that there was a 25 percent *lower* rate of prescription painkiller overdose deaths in those states. In other words, when people have a viable option to prescription painkillers, they are less likely to use prescription drugs and also less likely to die from overdosing on them.[34]

Lynne McTaggart, author of *What Doctors Don't Tell You: The Truth About the Dangers of Modern Medicine*, is a leading edge researcher and educator who promotes access to natural medicine. In a blog on her website McTaggart said:

> At the moment, as I have written earlier on these pages, conventional modern medicine kills thousands more people than it cures. Despite all the disingenuous attempts by "new" visitors to these pages to cast doubt about the quality of our research, there is no argument about the fact that modern

medicine remains the third deadliest killer in the West. No one in Establishment medicine disputes this.

Cochrane Collaboration co-founder and esteemed medical researcher Peter Goetzsche refers to the statistics in *Deadly Medicine and Organized Crime*, and it was first cited more than a decade ago by the *Journal of the American Medical Association*. At that time, said JAMA, medicine was ranked the fourth leading cause of death—since that time it's moved up in the league tables of things most likely to kill you.

That stat was first put forward by doctors and is now accepted as fact by doctors.

So we have a system of medicine that, by its own admission, kills more people than anything other than heart disease and cancer every year, and yet is carrying out a systematized attack on anything else that might actually work and work safely.

What this means is that modern medicine, infiltrated and now run by the pharmaceutical industry, is attempting to deny you access to safe and effective health care. That, to my mind, is a violation of your basic human rights. In fact it is essentially a form of persecution—no less than it was to deny a black in the pre-1960 American South a seat on the bus.

What are we to do about this in a positive way? We can take the lead from Iceland, where a group of 500 concerned citizens launched Heilsufrelsi (Health Freedom), a new health freedom association, to ensure that natural medicine is safeguarded and Icelanders have access to natural ways of maintaining their health.

The new organization (http://www.heilsufrelsi.is), which was embraced by numerous doctors as well as patients, has pledged to start a dialogue with the island's medical establishment in order to ensure a "mature" and "rational" exchange and the shift toward, as speaker Dr Gunnar Rafn put it, "empathic, patient-centred, integrative medicine".

Instead of acting like an oppressed minority or continuing to play a game with loaded dice, it is now time for all of us interested in natural health care to unabashedly stand up for natural health freedom, organize together and insist on that mature dialogue.[35]

In one recent year there were 225,000 deaths in the United States that were attributed to iatrogenic causes. They included 12,000 deaths due to unnecessary surgery, 7,000 due to medication errors in hospitals, 20,000 due to other errors in hospitals, 80,000 due to infections in hospitals, and 106,000 due to non-error, negative effects of drugs.[36] Those are shocking numbers—but they are even more shocking when we consider that this study only addressed the deaths from iatrogenic causes in the U.S. How many people are impacted around the world?

Considering that cannabis may have helped many of them, wouldn't it be wonderful if it had been available to these patients? And what if the average doctor prescribed it and if it was also administered in hospitals? How many of those patients might still be alive if that were the case? I long for the day when everyone is afforded the options of medicinal cannabis and other alternative medicines and treatments if that is their preference.

Chapter 6

Which Sub-Species Do You Prefer—Sativa for *Energizing* or Indica for *Relaxing*?

There are two main sub-species or strains of the cannabis plant—sativa and indica. However, not all cannabis products are labeled as sativa or indica since many of the strains today are hybrids that contain attributes of both. **Many—if not most—of today's edible cannabis products are not designated as either sativa or indica, so if you're primarily interested in the edibles you may want to skip this short chapter.**

Within the sub-species of cannabis sativa and cannabis indica there are hundreds of different specific strains, each of which has its own unique name and its own unique chemical makeup. A recent web search came up with strains called Stonehedge, Black Gold, White Lightning, Strawberry Kush, and Pitbull, among many, many others.

If you are buying a product that's labeled as either sativa or indica, it's helpful to understand the main qualities of both of these sub-species because, in most cases, they provide the guidelines for *when* to use that particular cannabis product. *Sativa* is generally chosen for its *energizing* qualities and used at a time of day when you want and need to be awake, alert, and energized—and when bedtime is at least six to eight hours away. *Indica* is *relaxing* and is therefore generally used in the evening or at bedtime. However, these are general guidelines and do not apply to all patients.

Sativa is considered to be good for depression, and therefore it's possible that a person who is depressed might benefit from the use of sativa exclusively. But if you're dealing with pain and nausea, an indica dominant strain may be the preferred choice. Also, for some people, sativa leads to the infamous "munchies," while indica strains can have *weight loss* effects for some people and *weight gain* effects for others, depending on what homeostasis means for each specific body.

Also, there are rare cases in which some people seem to be "switched," which means that they have an opposite reaction: sativa is relaxing and indica is energizing. It's not common but it can and does happen. The switching may be caused by the person's body chemistry or their own unique health condition. On those occasions when I experimented with sativa during the day, I found that it heightened one of my symptoms, wobbliness, while indica seemed to quell some other symptoms a bit and did not cause me to be more wobbly. For that reason, I no longer take sativa at all.

The best way to check on whether you might react to indica or sativa in an opposite way from most others is to take the cannabis earlier than usual. For example, if you take an indica strain on a day when you can go to sleep early if your body wants to, the worst case scenario is that you take it at six in the evening—and then, when it kicks in, you go to bed super-early. But you wouldn't lose a night's sleep if it gives you the opposite effect. Similarly, if you take sativa in the morning when you don't have to drive or do anything that's important, and you find that it relaxes you instead of energizing you, you can take a long nap.

While I'm on the subject of people whose reactions to cannabis are "switched," dosage is another arena in which people can have vastly different reactions. Despite the fact that it seems totally counter-intuitive, some thin people require much larger doses of cannabis than heavier people. That's why starting slowly and building your dosage is so important.

As I mentioned earlier, since more and more strains of cannabis are being produced now that contain *both* indica and sativa qualities, many of the cannabis products available today are NOT labeled as one or the other. So if you don't see the designation of either sativa or indica on a product, it is almost assuredly a hybrid that contains both.

Chapter 7

Why the Strain of Medical Marijuana That You Take Matters

Now let's look at the complex chemistry of the cannabis plant. Nature has lavished each strain of the plant with anywhere between 400 and 500 chemical compounds, all of which work together synergistically. It's the ratio of these chemicals that gives each strain its own unique chemical profile, which fall into three main categories:

1. ***Terpenes*** are responsible for the distinct odor of cannabis
2. ***Flavonoids*** contribute color to the plant
3. ***Cannabinoids*** are believed to be responsible for the greatest medicinal value

Currently, when selecting a product, we focus mostly on the cannabinoid content, which consists of 80 to 100 different specific cannabinoids including THC and CBD. However, as more research is done on the terpenes and flavonoids, we are likely to learn a great deal more about their unique qualities and the roles they play in the entourage effect for patients.

The process of creating new strains of cannabis and determining which ones are the most beneficial for different health challenges is painstaking and time-consuming. However, these "new," more medicinal strains aren't really new; in a way, we're just rediscovering or recreating them. Medical cannabis pioneer Patrick Lang explains why it can take five to ten years to create a new, stable healing strain:

> Strain development is one of the most time-consuming processes in the development of medical cannabis. It takes great expertise and can easily take five to ten years to produce a stabilized strain from seed. Most of today's hybrids are one-offs produced by indoor cultivators who have a proven female strain (cultivated from mother plants and clones; clones are the indoor standard) and pollen from a male seedling plant, usually produced by an outdoor cultivator. They cross the two, wait for seeds to form, then plant the seeds and see if anything of great interest results. Typically 20% of the seeds will have the same chemical profile as the mother, 20% like the father, and 60% is a combination of both. It is in the 60% where unique strains come from. Each plant has to mature before it can be tested and then it gets pricey quickly. Testing a cross breed for its chemical composition costs $50 for THC and CBD alone. And when additional tests are added to determine the profile of other potentially valuable molecules, costs escalate. If we test 100 plants for THC and CBD alone at $50 per plant, the cost is $5,000. It is easy to see how the costs add up, especially considering multiple tests on each plant. Indoor cultivators don't care about seeds, so they sometimes get lucky with a one-off strain, but it can be challenging to preserve one-off strains with medically effective molecular profiles if you don't have stabilized seeds.[37]

Prior to the marijuana prohibition in the U.S. in the 1930s, cannabis was a commonly used medication, carried in most doctor's medical bags, and listed in pharmacology textbooks. However, it's likely that the cannabis medicines of that era had a low ratio of THC, which is responsible for psychoactive reactions such as feelings of euphoria, distorted or enhanced perception, or a high or stoned feeling. In fact, it's possible that the cannabis of that era had such a low THC level that patients experienced little to no psychoactivity.

After cannabis was made illegal, the THC level in most cannabis was dramatically increased due to "market" demands. Growers started altering the strains that were available, breeding "super weed" strains that contained higher and higher amounts of THC so less was needed to get high. Some experts believe that most of the illegal marijuana sold on the streets in recent years contained a THC content that's between *10 and 25 times more potent* than it was only a few decades ago. Other sources believe that those numbers may be inflated; however, even if that's the case, it's obvious that the illegal street market has been focused on extremely high-THC strains. That's unfortunate for those of us who are focused on the medicinal qualities because, while they were breeding plants which provided vastly more THC, the new strains they created had much lower amounts of other compounds such as CBD that are credited with many healing properties. In fact, some of the high-THC strains propagated by the illegal trade have *almost no* CBD. That doesn't mean that a strain that contains mostly THC isn't healing; however, it may be much less healing than other strains that contain more of the other cannabinoids.

Today's medical marijuana growers are attempting to breed strains that are like the strains that were used for medicine long ago. The only problem, as one expert explained to me, is this: "We really don't know the chemical makeup of those strains from decades and decades ago. Nobody knows the best ratio of THC, CBD, and other cannabinoids for various health challenges. We just have to experiment until we come up with strains that are the best for healing, which is a time-consuming and painstaking process."[38]

Each of the 80 to 100 individual cannabinoids in any specific cannabis plant has its own unique properties and qualities. The number of cannabinoids in any one plant ranges from 80 to 100 because each strain of cannabis has its own unique chemical profile, with some cannabinoids present in very tiny amounts and others not present at all. Also, some of the cannabinoids that are present in very minute quantities in the raw plant are destroyed when it goes through processing.

The two cannabinoids that you will hear the most about are tetrahydrocannabinol (THC) and cannabidiol (CBD) because these two cannabinoids are found in the highest quantities in most cannabis strains:

> **Tetrahydrocannabinol (THC)** is, by far, the cannabinoid that stands out the most because it's the chemical that produces the psychoactive high and feelings of euphoria associated with cannabis; therefore, the more THC contained in the plant, the more psychoactive it will be. THC is associated with these benefits: relieves pain and inflammation, reduces vomiting and nausea, suppresses muscle spasms, inhibits cell growth in tumors and cancer cells, and has antioxidant activity. For many patients, it also stimulates the appetite, which is very helpful to those who are undergoing treatments that cause a lack of appetite. (Note: THC is NOT present in cannabis that has not been heated; see "THCa" below for an understanding of this non-psychoactive precursor to THC.)
>
> **Cannabidiol (CBD)** is the cannabinoid that many medical marijuana experts are focused on today because it is considered to be one of the most medicinally therapeutic

compounds in the plant. CBD relieves pain, inflammation, anxiety, coughs, congestion, nausea and vomiting; it kills bacteria or slows its growth, reduces blood sugar levels, reduces seizures and convulsions, suppresses muscle spasms, reduces the risks of artery blockages, inhibits cell growth in tumors and cancer cells, treats psoriasis, promotes bone growth, tranquilizes (as a schizophrenia and psychosis management tool), reduces contractions in the small intestines, and protects nervous system degeneration. High-CBD cannabis may benefit patients with many different health problems, including anxiety, multiple sclerosis, and Tourette syndrome. Many new products that are high in CBD are now available—and, as with many aspects of cannabis medicine, there is not a universal perspective on how to label them. However, the website http://ProjectCBD.org gives the following suggestion for terminology that distinguishes between **CBD-rich** and **CBD dominant** strains: "By 'CBD-rich,' we mean a cannabis strain or product that has equal amounts of CBD and THC, or more CBD than THC (usually at least 4 percent CBD by dry weight.). By 'CBD-dominant,' we mean strains or products that are CBD-rich but have very little THC content."[39] For patients who are seeking high-CBD strains, some products are now being labeled by the ratio of CBD to THC in their chemical profiles. For example, a product that is labeled as "CBD 2:1" contains two times the amount of CBD to THC. While some of the therapeutic benefits of CBD are also attributed to THC, as with all of the chemical compounds in cannabis, the synergy or so-called entourage effect of all of the chemicals working together is also at play.

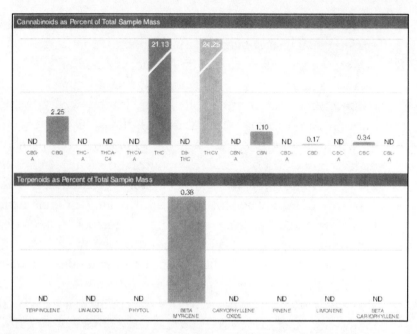

This illustration shows the percentage of cannabinoids and terpenoids in a specific strain of cannabis. Note that the top section lists 15 cannabinoids and the percentage of each—and that 9 of the cannabinoids listed are not present in a detectible trace amount (ND) in this sample. The bottom half of the chart, which charts the terpenes (also called terpenoids), indicates that only one of eight terpenoids commonly found in cannabis are present in this sample.[40]

When you see a cannabinoid abbreviation with an "a" at the end, the "a" stands for the word "acid." The "acid form" of any cannabinoid is **present only when cannabis is raw.** For example, let's look at the raw acid form of the most common cannabinoid, THC:

> **Tetrahydrocannabinolic acid (THCa):** Usually the main compound in raw cannabis, THCa is the biosynthetic precursor of THC. THCa does NOT cause psychoactivity; it converts to regular THC *only* when dried or heated for a period of time or burned or vaporized. If it's not heated, it is

still THCa. THCa has anti-inflammatory and neuroprotective effects. As I mentioned earlier, there is a growing "raw" cannabis movement. In part, that's because of the lack of psychoactivity in raw cannabis, but also because some experts believe it is a superior way to ingest cannabis due to unique healing properties it contains. There are three main types of raw cannabis products: 1) raw cannabis that's juiced and mixed with other juices to make it more palatable or even included in green salads; 2) cannabis oil that's manufactured through a cold-processing method and is available in capsules and syringes, among other types of products; or 3) low dose whole plant tablets made with raw cannabis. I'll give more specifics on raw cannabis products later.

Among the other cannabinoids that have been studied for their healing properties, here are a few more that stand out:

Cannabinol (CBN) is a therapeutic cannabinoid that relieves pain, aids sleep, and suppresses muscle spasms.

Cannabigerol (CBG) is like CBD in that it is not psychoactive; it is beneficial in killing or slowing bacteria growth, reducing inflammation, inhibiting cell growth in tumors and cancer cells, and promoting bone growth. CBG is also helpful in the treatment of glaucoma because it helps to relieve intraocular pressure.

Cannabichromene (CBC) is beneficial in pain relief, reduces inflammation, inhibits cell growth in tumors and cancer cells, is anti-microbial, and promotes bone growth.

Cannabichromene Acid (CBC-A) is believed to possess anti-inflammatory, antibacterial, and antifungal activity.

Tetrahydrocannabivarin (THCV) suppresses appetite, helps with weight loss, reduces seizures and convulsion, and promotes bone growth.

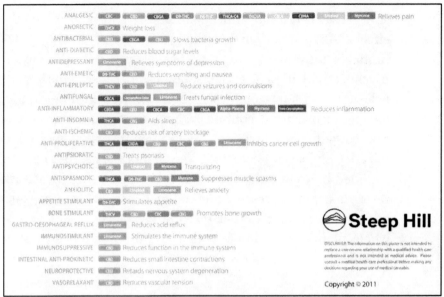

This chart from Steep Hill Lab[41] lists the prime benefits of some of the most-studied cannabinoids and terpenes.

As I mentioned, the cannabinoids that are specifically mentioned here are only a small number of the 80 to 100 that are found in any one cannabis plant. Most medical cannabis experts believe it is likely that every one of them plays a beneficial role, no matter how small the quantity might be. An article on the Steep Hill Lab website explains more about the ongoing study of cannabinoids, some of which show up in extremely tiny amounts in the plant:

> In genus Cannabis, most cannabinoids are present only in very tiny amounts, making identification and characterization a slow process. As a result, little is known about the chemical and physical properties unique to each of these chemical compounds. Currently, the cannabinoids found in highest concentration (through selective hybridization) and therefore

most studied are THC-A, CBD-A, CGB-A, and THCV-A, along with their neutral forms, THC, CBD, CBG and THCV. Recently strains rich in CBC-A have become more readily available for investigation; it was recently reported in a study that CBC is ten times more potent in managing stress than CBD, requiring 1/10 as much to obtain the same result as with CBD.[42]

What we know for sure is that, in many ways, medical cannabis research is still in its infancy. Large pharmaceutical companies are researching the healing qualities of specific cannabinoids so they can develop new drugs by creating synthetic versions of them. Concurrently, medical marijuana experts, most of whom believe that *all* of the cannabinoids have a role to play in healing, are using the same scientific data to come up with new strains that are targeted to benefit patients with specific diseases and health issues. In the paragraph from Steep Hill Lab that I quote above I'm intrigued by the last sentence: "... it was recently reported in a study that CBC is ten times more potent in managing stress than CBD ...." That's fascinating because CBC is one of the least known chemicals in cannabis and yet scientists have clearly identified unique and important virtues that are imparted by it.

That same article on the Steep Hill Lab website also discusses research on another cannabinoid, THCV, which is being found to be highly effective in treating post-traumatic stress disorder (PTSD).

These are just two examples of the type of specialized research that's focused on specific cannabinoids. As scientists and growers research and study each individual cannabinoid and its specific healing qualities, they continue to use that knowledge to breed and grow new strains of cannabis with specific health issues in mind.

When you look for the quantity of each of the cannabinoids in a specific product online or on the packaging itself, generally you will find very limited information. Some products list only the quantity of THC; others also include CBD and CBN. Looking at the chemical profiles of a number of cannabis products on a recent Internet search, I chose a few examples that will give you a better idea of how widely the quantity of THC, CBD, and CBN ranges from product to product. I've created two charts—one for high-THC products and the other for high-CBD products.

High-THC Products
Cannabinoid Content

	THC	CBD	CBN
Product #1	58.59%	0.92%	0.53%
Product #2	45.18%	1.66%	0.14%
Product #3	20.32%	0.07%	0.00%
Product #4	41.76%	0.18%	0.00%

These four high-THC products show a wide range in the ratio of cannabinoids from one strain to the next and they all have a low CBD content that's under 1%. Note that the last two products list the CBN content as 0%.

Here are some ratios of high-CBD products listed on the same website:

High-CBD Products
Cannabinoid Content

	THC	CBD	CBN
Product #5	5.39%	50.66%	0.19%
Product #6	28.35%	52.77%	0.09%
Product #7	6.74%	14.54%	0.00%
Product #8	35.54%	36.18%	0.25%

Again, this group of products shows quite a range in the amount of each cannabinoid that's in a specific strain and also quite a range on the ratios. The first product in the High-CBD product list has the lowest THC of all four (5.39%) and also a fairly high level of CBD (50.66%). Remember, there are between 80 and 100 cannabinoids in each strain of cannabis. It is the ratio of *all of the chemicals*, including the terpenes and flavonoids, that gives each strain its own unique chemical profile, making it almost like a different medicine from every other strain, with its own unique set of mechanisms to bring homeostasis to the body.

Chapter 8

How Marijuana Balances Your Autonomic Nervous System—And Why That's Important

Your body's autonomic nervous system *loves* balance and harmony—and many experts say that cannabis can assist with this in ways unlike any other medication. The autonomic nervous system regulates *automatic* functions in the body, such as breathing, blood pressure regulation, beating of the heart, functioning of the bladder, and digestion. Its two branches—the *sympathetic nervous system* and the *parasympathetic nervous system*—constantly work together to harmonize and balance the body.

The sympathetic nervous system deals with stress and the "fight, flight, or freeze" response that we deal with frequently in our fast-paced society. Many times during the day, as stresses appear, your sympathetic nervous system automatically kicks in and provides you with the tools that are needed to respond to those stresses. Even seemingly small decisions, such as the choice you make when you approach a yellow light at an intersection, is attended to by your sympathetic nervous system. In the split-second that you have to make a decision, you will either give the car a bit more gas when you come upon the yellow light or, instead, you might decide to put on the brakes. There's not much time to weigh your options; you have to

Norma Eckroate

respond very quickly to the stimuli around you. Then, after the stress is over, the parasympathetic nervous system kicks in and returns the body to a more regenerative and normal state of peace and relaxation. That's the best case scenario—and that's what happens when the body is operating efficiently. On the other side of the coin, when the body is frequently overtaxed and in a state of overwhelm, the tensions of imbalance mount up. If that happens on a fairly constant basis, the body is more vulnerable to illness and disease.

Joan Bello, researcher and author of *The Benefits of Marijuana*, beautifully explains the role marijuana plays with the autonomic nervous system in these two excerpts:

> When we balance the Autonomic Nervous System, there is an effect on the mind that is both energizing and relaxing SIMULTANEOUSLY. In other words, we can think more clearly and more efficiently.[43]
>
> The net effect is a highly functioning, yet relaxed, system with better fuel. This is why, with marijuana, the feeling is both relaxed and alert, which explains, in part, the experience of being "stoned." Normally the body vacillates between the two opposing modes of being. The effects of the complicated marijuana molecule somehow actually integrate these two modes, simultaneously, as absolutely nothing else does.[44]

In her book, Bello also reminds us that many pharmaceutical medications put the body into an altered state of **un**consciousness—a state of relaxation *without awareness*. Since my choice has always been to pursue holistic options as much as possible and allopathic drugs as a last resort, my experience with pharmaceutical drugs is not as extensive as that of most people who are my age. However, over the years, I still have taken enough powerful pharmaceuticals to have my own confirmation of Bello's point. Comparing marijuana to some of these pharmaceuticals, I realize that some of the drugs put me in a deep state of *unawareness*. On the other hand, the altered state of consciousness from marijuana causes *heightened awareness*, even while it also causes greater relaxation.

When the nervous system is overly stressed too often and for too long, it can become dysfunctional. In most cases, when this happens, the sympathetic nervous system remains dominant and the parasympathetic nervous system doesn't turn on—causing a constant state of fight, flight, or freeze. The autonomic nervous system's stress response, which is designed to deal with brief emergencies, isn't equipped to handle constant stress and the result is degeneration and dis-ease in the body.

Bello also explains marijuana's effect on the autonomic nervous system to enhance *both* sides of the brain. She says:

> Through its increased Sympathetic action, left brain perception is heightened while, at the same time, right brain reception is enhanced. This is a physiological fact. More blood, and cleaner blood, is sent to the brain, as in the "fight or flight" reaction. And because of Parasympathetic dilation of all capillaries, which signifies relaxation, the blood supply to the entire brain is increased. More blood means more oxygen and consequently clear and broader thinking. Since marijuana works on both sides of the brain, the most noticeable effect, in our fast-paced mind set, is one of slowing down, which blends the thrusting competitive attitude with the contrasting viewpoint of nurturance to arrive at a more cooperative balance. This experience is, however, not innate to marijuana, but to the mental state of the subject. When we are mellow, tired, and relaxed, marijuana is energizing and affords alertness, determination, and even strength. ... It both stimulates and relaxes, simultaneously, which equates to an unpredictable variation in effect that is solely dependent on the state of its subject. When the system is sluggish, as for

natives in warm climates (Africa, India, South America), marijuana has been used extensively and for centuries to energize it.[45]

I took special note of Bello's explanation that an individual's experience with cannabis is determined by their mental state at the time. Bello also explains that when the sympathetic and parasympathetic are balanced through the use of cannabis, balance is restored to the body in these ways:

- Muscles relaxed
- Pupils constricted
- Blood pressure slightly lowered
- Heart rate slightly raised
- Mucus membranes dry
- Bronchi dilated
- Veins and arteries dilated
- Breathing: Slow, Deep, Regular[46]

As I lay down to go to sleep at night, I often tune into my breathing and note that it has become deeper since I have been taking cannabis—leading to a greater depth of relaxation in my entire body. I give medical cannabis a lot of the credit for this because I know that it often leads to increased lung capacity. And, from a holistic perspective, I would be remiss if I didn't also share with you a breathing method I studied called Buteyko Breathing, which I also attribute to my improved lung capacity.[47]

So why is our breathing so important to our health? It's helpful to look at Bello's explanation of why breathing capacity improves for most people when they start taking cannabis. The alveoli (sacs in the lungs) expand, allowing for better elimination of stale air and increased oxygen intake, causing breathing to be slower and more expansive. And the rib cage also contributes because marijuana relaxes the skeletal muscles, including the muscles that constrain the ribs. In addition, the brain receives more blood due to dilation in the brain capillaries and the blood is more richly oxygenated. Then the heart rate rises slightly and that speeds up the distribution of this oxygenated blood in the body.[48]

Chapter 9

Why Your Body's Self-Healing System Works Better with Natural Methods and Products

One of the principles of holistic healing is that the body is programmed to deal with any challenges to its well-being by healing *itself* when provided with the right conditions. When it is given the raw materials that promote well-being, the body's self-healing system kicks into gear and responds to any condition or stimulus that is disruptive. Another way of saying this is that when a "disruption" occurs, the body does its best to maintain internal stability and equilibrium by triggering the physiological processes needed to achieve the harmony and balance of *homeostasis*.

Homeostasis Works on a Cellular Level

In his book, *The Science of Healing Revealed*, atomic medical physicist Dr. Gary Samuelson explains how homeostasis works on a cellular level when the cells have been damaged:

> ... in order for the body to heal itself, it must be able to detect and locate the damaged cells. This task goes to the cellular-

distress messengers. These messengers are sent out in response to a distress condition inside the cell. This distress condition occurs in the cell when something interferes with the normal cellular processes and disturbs the normal homeostatic chemical balance. This homeostatic chemical balance depends on the cell being able to constantly produce the thousands of critical molecules it needs and then being able to break them down at the same rate that they are being produced. When this balance is disturbed, certain molecules are either building up in the cell or becoming depleted. These excesses or deficiencies cause transcription-factor messengers to be sent into the DNA that change certain production rates that hopefully will ultimately compensate for the imbalance. Sometimes the response includes an increase in the amount of messengers sent out to signal this condition to other cells.[49]

The wisdom of the body is awesome and its desire for homeostasis is ever-constant—but when the body becomes overwhelmed, it can break down to a point of disease. Unfortunately, most doctors have not been trained to uncover, understand, and treat the imbalances that caused a disease in the first place, including emotional issues that may have played a role.

The allopathic medicine that most of doctors practice, which is focused on treating the symptoms of disease, often involves medications that can cause even more imbalances in the body. From the perspective of those who understand and practice holistic, body-mind-spirit wellness, the preferred choice is to use natural healing alternatives, which are focused on healing the causes of the body's disturbance. In fact, many leading edge doctors predict that today's standard allopathic medical treatments, some of which have dismal survival rates, will be viewed as barbaric by future generations.

Why Symptom Relief from Pharmaceutical Drugs Is Often Like a Band-Aid

In the book *Cannabis Chemotherapy*, David Hoye and his coauthors speak to the ways that pharmaceutical drugs often lead to more pharmaceutical drugs because, in most cases, *they are designed to deal only with symptoms, not to heal the cause of a health challenge*:

> In this country we don't get cures for health issues; we get symptom relief. This is what medical practice has essentially become—prescribing drugs in a five-minute session with your doctor, which is about all one can accomplish in five minutes. Got a health problem? Here's a drug for the symptoms. Got a side effect? Here's another drug for that. Got another side effect from that? No problem, here's another drug. Rarely are drugs exchanged one for another these days; they tend to be added. Has the problem been cured? No, it's been suppressed under all those drugs. And by this time it wouldn't be unusual to have all the side effects confused with yet another symptom of something else. And we know what the treatment for that will be.
>
> But wait, there's more. Sales of drugs for children have been the pharmaceutical industry's fastest growing business. Doctors now prescribe drugs to children for everything from high cholesterol to anxiety, not to mention ADHD. Pharmaceutical sales reps urge doctors to prescribe antidepressants, antipsychotics and other psychiatric meds to children. So our children now take three times more attention deficit and antidepressant drugs than children in Europe. It's unconscionable.[50]

Unlike more natural substances such as medicinal herbs, pharmaceutical drugs are designed to eliminate symptoms, they are *not* designed to treat the *cause* of health issues and actually repair the body. An excellent resource on holistic health is http://Shirleys-Wellness-Cafe.com, which includes this explanation for the prevalence of chronic illness in our modern world:

> Physicians and surgeons palliate symptoms instead of removing causes. The immune system is not responsive to drugs for healing. Antibiotics used to fight infections actually depress the immune system when used long-term. Standard Western Medicine strives to suppress the immune response, working against the body. If there is a fever, lower it, if inflammation is present provide steroids to remove it and of course if Western Medicine thinks a bacteria or virus is present or doesn't know what is wrong, a dose of anti-biotics is provided. This way of doing things can be effective in the immediate term, and important in life threatening situations, but potentially devastating in the long term especially when over-used. Because, what eventually happens, is that immune system becomes weak and ineffective or damaged and over-reactive and disease is pushed deeper into the body to come back stronger and more difficult to get rid of at a later date. This is called trading ACUTE disease for long-term CHRONIC disease, and it is one reason why so many of us are chronically ill today.[51]

Another concern with many pharmaceutical drugs is the possibility of becoming addicted to some of them. In the media, we hear many stories of people taking a drug for legitimate reasons, as prescribed by their doctors, and then, over time, become unwittingly addicted to it, and starting to use it illegally. Most people don't realize that those drugs can build up in the system and that they can also interact with each other. Even if a drug works well for you initially, its potential negative side effects can cause problems over time. Among the many possible symptoms of drug toxicity are memory loss, blurred vision, mental disorientation, dizziness, fainting, and falls.

The reasons a person may experience drug toxicity include:

- Interactions between a specific medication and other prescription drugs, over-the-counter medications, herbal medicines, and/or nutritional supplements.
- A new prescription from a doctor who hasn't been informed about medications that were prescribed by other doctors.
- The ability to metabolize a drug has diminished over time.
- When a new symptom is caused by drug interactions and, instead of identifying that as the cause, the doctor prescribes yet another medication for the "new" symptom.
- If the patient has lost weight, the dosage may be too high at the lower weight.
- The body's ability to eliminate drugs and other toxins through the kidneys and liver becomes progressively harder as a person ages; therefore, as their ability to do their jobs are diminished, our organs are less and less efficient—and our bodies become more toxic.

Cannabis to the Rescue for Children Too

As many of us reconsider everything that we thought we knew about cannabis, it's impossible to overlook reports of very sick children being healed or showing dramatic improvement from a number of conditions, including tumors and severe seizure disorders. These reports are showing up in articles and videos on mainstream media and the Internet in increasing numbers. In some of these cases, the child was treated with low- or non-psychoactive forms of cannabis such as very high-CBD strains or raw cannabis products.

When we think of the smallest and most vulnerable patients, it can get a bit tricky. In many of these cases, parents turned to cannabis as a last resort after every allopathic treatment and medication failed to help. As with so many issues surrounding this herb, it's difficult to find studies on the safety of cannabis for children because the U.S. government has made it almost impossible to conduct such studies. However, at least one study addressed the issue of how cannabis might impact the unborn fetus and the newborn. In her excellent book, *The Benefits of Marijuana*, researcher Joan Bello reviews a study that focused on the effects of cannabis use by pregnant women in Jamaica. Bello says:

> In Jamaica—where the stigma of marijuana is nearly nonexistent, a very meaningful study has been reported concerning women who ingested the herb while pregnant and the effects it had on the unborn fetus, as well as on the infants whose mothers continued to use marijuana while breast-feeding. The study was under the auspices of the University of Massachusetts Nursing Education Department and published in Pediatrics.
>
> The results were absolutely favorable for the marijuana-exposed babies when compared to the control group of non-exposed infants. This was not really a surprise considering the general health-giving benefits of Cannabis. Jamaica was the locale of preference, specifically because "Scientific reports have documented the cultural integration of marijuana and its ritual and medicinal, as well as recreational functions," thereby disallowing any bias that could contaminate the findings.[52]

Cannabis is a natural product that helps to stabilize physiological processes in the body, leading to homeostasis. It is considered to be an adaptogen, a term that is applied to some medicinal herbs, nutritional supplements, and foods that "adapt" to each body's unique needs to stimulate immunity and help the body regenerate after being stressed. Dr. Frank Lipman explains it this way:

> Adaptogens work a bit like a thermostat. When the thermostat senses that the room temperature is too high it brings it down; when the temperature is too low it brings it up. Adaptogens can calm you down and boost your energy at the same time without over stimulating. They can normalize body imbalances. By supporting adrenal function, they counteract the adverse effects of stress. They enable the body's cells to access more energy; help cells eliminate toxic byproducts of the metabolic process and help the body to utilize oxygen more efficiently. In short, adaptogens are amazing![53]

Because of the long track record of the safety and efficacy of cannabis as a natural, adaptogenic remedy, Joan Bello suggests that we open our minds to the ways in which it can help children. She says:

> As an adaptogenic remedy, there is no rationale for keeping the benefits of marijuana from infants, children, or teens. It's "usefulness" for the instabilities suffered so often episodically in youthful, vibrant organisms is unsurpassed. For the life-diminishing diseases, such as autism or other non-treatable problems that usually are diagnosed in early childhood, the benefits of Marijuana Therapy are just beginning to emerge via parents who have utilized marijuana as a last resort— which fortunately revitalized their hopes by affecting their children extremely favorably.[54]

Some doctors who are proponents of medical cannabis for adults still question whether it is safe to treat children with cannabis, citing concerns about how it might impact a child's developing brain. However, when no other treatment works and the child is in desperate straits, even those doctors agree that cannabis should be given to the child.

Other doctors see no reason NOT to treat children with cannabis because the evidence of its multitude of benefits is solid. On the video *Cannabis Rising,* Dr. Lester Grinspoon, Emeritus Professor of Psychiatry at Harvard Medical School is asked, "How young is too young to use medicinal marijuana?" Dr. Grinspoon responded:

> How young is too young to use aspirin? How young is too young to use penicillin? I can't guarantee it's going to do anything but I can tell you it isn't going to harm him. It is remarkably non-toxic. We have been brainwashed about this substance. There will come a time when people will recognize that this is a wonder drug of our times. It does so much in terms of relieving some of the symptoms which are very difficult for parents to deal with—let alone the child.[55]

Dr. William Courtney, who pioneered the use of fresh, raw cannabis juice to treat his patients, says he successfully treated an eight-month-old baby for a brain tumor. Here is part of a HuffPost Live interview in which this baby's case is discussed with Dr. Courtney:

> Medical marijuana is gaining acceptance, but could it even help kids? Dr. William Courtney has seen it happen, and on Friday, told HuffPost Live host Alyona Minkovski about it. Saying he was "quite a skeptic 5 or 6 years ago," Dr. Courtney continued that "my youngest patient is 8 months old, and had a very massive centrally located inoperable brain tumor." The child's father pushed for non-traditional treatment utilizing cannabis.

They were putting cannabinoid oil on the baby's pacifier twice a day, increasing the dose.... And within two months there was a dramatic reduction, enough that the pediatric oncologist allowed them to go ahead with not pursuing traditional therapy.

The tumor was remarkably reduced after eight months of treatment. Dr. Courtney pointed out that the success of the cannabis approach means that "this child, because of that, is not going to have the long-term side effects that would come from a very high dose of chemotherapy or radiation... currently the child's being called a miracle baby, and I would have to agree that this is the perfect response that we should be insisting is frontline therapy for all children before they launch off on all medications that have horrific long term side effects."[56]

Balancing the Benefits of Integrative Medicine Versus Allopathic Medicine

Today there are more and more practitioners of integrative medicine, which is also referred to as complementary and alternative medicine (CAM), natural medicine, and a few other labels, who integrate holistic health modalities in their practices. For many years I have followed the books, seminars, and interviews of top holistic medical doctors and other alternative practitioners. They have divergent opinions on some topics—and, in general, they are not fans of most allopathic medicine—but they all say the same thing when it comes to traumatic injuries: "If I get hit by a car, please take me to an emergency room and make sure they give me everything they have to put me back together again." You see, most integrative practitioners agree that modern Western medicine does a really *good* job in dealing with trauma.

Drugs and surgeries are welcome when they are the first line of defense for a mangled, bleeding body—and that's also the case when some life-threatening conditions arise, such as heart attacks and strokes. But how did we get to the point where physicians prescribe drugs that are later taken off the market because they were actually dangerous? Just have a look at the website of any law firm that specializes in personal injury lawsuits. Prominent on those websites you will see a long list of drugs and medical devices that were, at some point in time, considered "safe" and approved by the Food and Drug Administration, only to be recalled after many injuries and deaths. Here's a question that I'd like you to consider: How can you be sure the drugs in use today are safer than those that were on the market for years and then—after injuries and even death occurred—taken off the market?

Clearly, the more natural the medicine, the less concern we need to have about a negative impact from it. The bottom line is that healing is very personal. When the body breaks down, we are often overwhelmed with the choices and decisions we have to make. That's why it's important to muster all of the resources and make choices that feel right to us. I believe that tapping into the incredible power of the mind is vital to the process.

I personally know five people who would be dead or at very least severely disabled today, except for the fact that they believe in miracles and they allowed a miracle of healing. Four of them are good friends and the fifth is a man I chatted with after hearing him give a talk. These healings range from decades ago to a few years ago. When I refer to their recoveries as miracles of healing, that's the way I see it. I know of people who credit prayer and the power of the mind for their healing and others who have used natural, alternative treatments, as well as many who have done both. It's all miraculous to me! As far as I know, none of them used medical cannabis, which is definitely not your only option to achieve greater wellness. However, it is an option that has helped so very many and one for which I am extremely appreciative.

Chapter 10

Why Emotional Healing is a Requirement for Physical Healing

Many doctors have treated patients who had "terminal" conditions—and were shocked when they *fully recovered*. And they have experienced the opposite too—patients for whom a full recovery was expected, but they died. It's certainly possible that the patients who died when their doctors expected a recovery had a more severe condition than the doctor was able to ascertain or even an undiagnosed secondary condition that contributed to their deaths. However, I believe a major factor in these outcomes is the emotional healing that the patient did—or did not—experience along the way.

The Critical Role of Emotional Health in Well-being

The science of *psychoneuroimmunology* is the study of the ways our health is impacted by our emotional state. Canadian physician, public speaker, and award-winning author, Gabor Maté, MD, incorporates the relatively new science of psychoneuroimmunology into his medical practice. In his book, *When the Body Says No: Exploring the Stress-Disease Connection*, Dr. Maté explains that "the internal milieu of thoughts and unconscious emotions" have a direct role in our physical well-being:

> This book shows that people do not become ill despite their lives but because of their lives. And life includes not only physical factors like diet, physical activity and the environment, but also the internal milieu of thoughts and unconscious emotions that govern so much of our physiology through the mechanisms of stress and the unity of the systems that modulate nerves, hormones, immunity, digestion, and cardiovascular function. Much disease could be prevented and healed if we fully understood the scientific evidence verifying the mind-body unity.[57]

Another leading edge doctor who is connecting the dots on the ways the health of the body is impacted by the mind is Lissa Rankin, MD. In her PBS television special, *Heal Yourself: Mind Over Medicine with Lissa Rankin*, the doctor explains the powerful role your mind plays in your well-being:

> You are the gatekeeper of your mind. You are responsible for your thoughts, beliefs, and feelings, which are critical when it comes to your health. The scientific data proves that your thoughts, beliefs, and feelings affect the physiology of your body more profoundly than you may realize. Now I get that that's a big statement. But think of it this way: You wouldn't take a pill with a skull and crossbones on it. Right? But I want you to understand that every negative thought that you have is poison for your body. Every pessimistic thought, every negative health belief, every angry feeling, every time you feel lonely, or resentful, or depressed. If you are stressed at work

or unhappy in your marriage, you are potentially harming your body. And every time you think optimistically or feel supported by a community of people or you get in touch with your life's purpose or your spiritual self, you are healing your body. This is a huge part of how you can be pro-active about taking back your health.[58]

Those quotes from Dr. Maté and Dr. Rankin are so powerful that I suggest reading them again and then returning to this paragraph. I often refer to the old, negative and limited thoughts, beliefs, feelings, and emotions that Dr. Maté and Dr. Rankin are referring to as "flawed premises." These flawed premises are held within the body and the consciousness—and they can keep us stuck in a lower emotional set-point for years or decades. To take responsibility for that which is holding us back, we can consciously *decide* to constantly monitor our thoughts on just about every topic, including our finances, relationships, and health.

As we gradually, bit by bit, release those thoughts, beliefs, feelings and emotions that have limited us for all or much of our lives, we lift our consciousness and metaphorically step onto the higher ground of a less judgmental, more loving, and more abundant life. We have to *want* to feel better by making emotional well-being a priority and consciously working toward that goal—and from that more aligned place the body is more empowered to heal itself.

Another pioneer, Dr. Mario Martinez, is a neuropsychologist who now refers to the field of psychoneuroimmunology as *biocognition.* Breaking down that word, the *bio* part relates to biology or the physical self, while *cognition* is how we think about things. In his decades of research, Dr. Martinez has discovered that all emotional wounds fit into at least one of three categories—shame, betrayal, and abandonment—although he explains that more than one of these categories can be at play simultaneously. Dr. Martinez explains that each of type of wounding causes an immunological response within the body and that these woundings are usually inflicted by people who are important in our lives and have authority over us. The woundings can be as simple as a child being rejected by another child in the playground or as complex as being spurned by a loved one.

The woundings keep the mind stuck in limited or negative thinking, which it repeats over and over and over, negatively impacting the immune system. They can be as simple as a child being rejected by another child in the playground or as complex as being spurned by a loved one.

As we heal the woundings that led to the feelings of shame, betrayal, or abandonment, Dr. Martinez says we free the mind and are then able to tap into greater well-being. Dr. Martinez has an excellent CD album and book, both of which are titled *The Mind-Body Code*. The subtitle of the CD album—*How the Mind Wounds and Heals the Body*—beautifully expresses the good news: The same mind that wounds the body also has the amazing ability to heal it. But, to do so, we have to let go of our sloppy thinking and focus more consistently on better feeling thoughts.

On the album, Dr. Martinez says that repressed emotions have desensitized most of us to the point that we don't even know that we're miserable. He calls this a "comfortable misery" because we are so used to it, and explains that, at a young age, we all learned "scripts of deprivation" from authority figures, which are actually negative beliefs that we've held onto:

> The people who have authority around you taught you the scripts of deprivation. "Your dad never made it; you're never going to make it." "You're not smart enough." "You're not good at this; you're not good at that." Although you think that you have gotten rid of them, and though you think you've overcome them, they are still part of your biology and need to be modified. The scripts of sabotage and the scripts of deprivation need to be addressed.[59]

Why Placebo Studies Prove the Power of Our Minds

The power of the mind to control the body has been documented by medical science for most of the past century. That's why scientists and researchers use double-blind placebo-controlled procedures in their studies. Because they know that people often experience outcomes that they subconsciously *expect* to experience, their goal is to make their studies as free from subjective bias as possible. For that reason, the studies are set up so neither the researchers nor the participants know who received a "real" substance and who received the "dummy" or inert substance, which is referred to as a placebo.

Just as the researchers who do placebo studies understand that the mind can empower or disempower any substance or treatment, we can intentionally do our best to line up our thinking whether we're exploring cannabis or something else. A study that dramatically speaks to the power of the placebo is detailed in Marc David's book, *The Slow Down Diet*. While David's book is focused on our psychological relationship with food, the fascinating double-blind placebo-controlled study he references in this excerpt was for a chemotherapy drug:

> In 1983, medical researchers were testing a new chemotherapy treatment. One group of cancer patients received the actual drug being tested while another group received a placebo—a fake, harmless, inert chemical substance. As you may know, pharmaceutical companies are required by law to test all new drugs against a placebo to determine the true effectiveness, if any, of the product in question. In the course of this study, no one thought twice when 74 percent of the cancer patients receiving the real chemotherapy exhibited one of the more common side effects of this treatment: they lost their hair. Yet, quite remarkably, 31 percent of the patients on the placebo chemotherapy—an

inert saltwater injection—also had an interesting side effect: they lost their hair too. Such is the power of expectation. The only reason that those placebo patients lost their hair is because they believed they would. Like many people, they associated chemotherapy with going bald.[60]

As the study participants apparently knew, hair loss is a common side effect of chemotherapy. However, as Marc David tells us, the only explanation for 31 percent of the patients who were taking the placebo to lose their hair is that they believed they were on the actual chemotherapy drug. That belief trumped the fact that they were not actually receiving the drug—and it caused their hair to fall out even though they were simply getting saltwater injections, not the chemotherapy drug.

Another interesting placebo study was conducted on a segment of an ABC television show called "Would You Fall for That?" It wasn't a long, elaborate double-blind study such as those the pharmaceutical companies set up; instead, it was an easy and quick demonstration that was designed to show the placebo effect in action. On the show, beach-goers were invited to take part in an "energy challenge." First, participants were asked to swing a mallet to test their strength on a carnival game called the High Striker. After one hit with the mallet to determine a baseline of their strength, contestants were told that a new "energy" drink was being tested and they were asked to drink a small bottle of it. What the contestants didn't know is that the bottle contained club soda, not a fancy new energy drink. After drinking the contents of the bottle, they were asked to strike the mallet again. And, of course, they all got a higher score—because they *believed* that they just drank something that gave them more energy and enabled them to hit the High Striker with more force.

This TV show experiment demonstrates something that many of us do all the time. When we believe in something, we automatically give it more power. When we *disbelieve* in something, we automatically *disempower* it. Because the power of our belief about any medicine or therapy can be important to its efficacy, aligning our thoughts and beliefs about it adds a layer of extra potency to the equation. But if we question a medicine or therapy, we are doing the opposite and aligning our thoughts and beliefs with it being *less effective.*

Just as the contents of the bottles seemingly took on magical properties when the participants believed they were drinking an energy drink, when we consciously align our thoughts and beliefs with what we want, what we believe manifests in our lives *because* we believe it. Of course, the same is true for the 31 percent of the participants who lost hair in the chemotherapy trial even though they were taking the placebo; they believed they were taking the real drug and their bodies responded to that message from their consciousness.

The concept of placebos can be summed up in one statement, "It is done unto you as you believe." Because of the power of the mind, it's impossible to totally isolate any treatment or supplement to determine how well it works since each person's alignment with that treatment or supplement *in the moment* has a big impact on its efficacy. The bottom line is that the power of the mind has a huge role in ANY healing—in fact, many experts believe it's the biggest factor. Therefore, your own healing is impacted by your answer to one primary question, *Do you want to get well?*

Our minds are powerful, whether we direct their focus or not. We can use our knowledge of the placebo effect in a positive way by focusing on and believing in the healing power of the modalities we chose to pursue so they are as effective as they can possibly be. The patients who have the best opportunity for improving their conditions are the ones who are willing to let go of the idea that they are powerless and, instead, step into their own empowerment.

The Importance of *Authentic* Affirmations

As you step into the awareness that flawed premises may have led to your illness in the first place—or at least contributed to it—insights will pop into your mind on this subject. Just be light about it. As negative or limiting thoughts pop into your conscious awareness, your goal is to gently stop in your tracks and identify them as flawed premises or beliefs. Say to yourself, "Wait a minute. I want to change that thought/belief. What feels better?" Then turn the flawed premise around. Here's how to do it: When you step into better feeling thoughts, it's imperative that those thoughts are authentic for you *in that very instant.* If your body feels sick and you say, "I am vibrantly healthy," your entire being knows that that affirmation is not true for you. And, guess what, saying an affirmation that resonates in your beingness as untrue makes you feel worse! That's the opposite of healing because whenever you say or do anything that makes you *feel* bad, your entire body chemistry is negatively impacted.

It's imperative to find better feeling thoughts that are authentic *for you* in the moment. So, as an example, instead of saying "I am vibrantly healthy," which may not align with the way you are feeling at that moment in time, find a positive statement you do believe in the moment. For example, you might say, "I know that some people have been healed from this condition; if they did it, *maybe* I can too." Some people might suggest that the word "maybe" in that sentence is too conditional for a proper affirmation. But if "*maybe* I can too" is the best you can do in the moment, then it's a great statement for you because being authentic in your statement is what's most important. Then, as you continue to work this inner dialogue process and start to ferret out the flawed premises that are causing limitations in your life, you will come to a point when you can authentically say, "I know that some people have been healed from this condition; if they did it, *I will too!*"

As you become aware of the flawed premises that have been running the operating system that is your mind-body and take action to step into a higher vibration of thought, you are also aligning with your true nature of wellness. And that will align you with the homeostasis that is always there for you, bringing greater harmony and balance—physically, mentally, and spiritually.

For more on emotional healing, I suggest that you tap into the ever-growing field of energy psychology, which offers leading edge methods such as Emotional Freedom Techniques (EFT), Matrix Energetics, and a number of others. For more information about energy psychology, see the website for the Association for Comprehensive Energy Psychology at http://www.energypsych.org.

Chapter 11

Every Patient's Question About Cannabis—
Will It Help Me?

When it comes to medical cannabis, the question that's most important to each patient is this: *Will it help me?* When we know for a fact that others were helped by cannabis, we are encouraged that it may help us too. And that is especially the case when we know that some of them have dealt with symptoms or conditions like those that are now challenging us.

This chapter is a bit of a review; however, we will also dig a bit deeper on the attributes of the chemical compounds in cannabis and the benefits they impact individually and collectively. We discussed the chemical compounds called cannabinoids in Chapter 7, and focused on the specific health benefits of a handful of those that have been studied the most, including the ways in which these compounds promote wellness in the body. But please remember that it's not just that handful of cannabinoids that provide health benefits. It's probable that ALL of the hundreds of cannabinoids and other chemical compounds in cannabis work together synergistically and that the maximum benefit comes from the entire array of cooperative components that Nature put in there.

While pharmaceutical drugs are designed to target specific symptoms, holistic remedies such as cannabis work in an intrinsic way on a cellular level. As you've learned in this book, there are between 400 and 500 chemical compounds in cannabis and, depending on the specific strain, up to 100 of them are cannabinoids. Different cannabis products, made from different strains of plants, affect the body differently because the percentage of chemical compounds in each product is different. And it's the ratio of each chemical relative to each of the others that determines each strain's characteristics and its healing qualities.

When people ask me if medical cannabis would be helpful for condition X or condition Y, I tell them, "It's my opinion that cannabis helps with almost anything." I tell them that because, as I said earlier, cannabis promotes homeostasis by working with the body's own endocannabinoid system to harmonize and balance all of the functions of the body. Does that mean that cannabis will help with symptom relief or even possibly lead to healing for any condition? As I said, I believe, at the very least, it can help. And that's especially the case when patients have access to strain(s) that are known to assist with symptoms and conditions they are dealing with.

You can probably guess that I also believe anyone who has conquered a challenging or life-threatening condition has also stepped into some degree of emotional healing on some level of their consciousness—or the physical healing wouldn't have happened. Therefore, I don't think any physical medication or treatment is ever the sole reason for healing. However, when we consider the crucially important role of the placebo effect, as discussed in Chapter 10, we also understand the importance of our own beliefs, since that's the way placebos work. When we believe that the medications and treatments we are receiving are going to help and we also believe in the wisdom of the health professionals who are guiding us on the journey, we might more easily jump ahead in our healing journey.

In an article for *US News*, Dr. William Courtney, a leading pioneer in the use of medical cannabis, listed just some of the attributes of the many chemical compounds in cannabis. He said:

The cannabinoid acids in cannabis have been found to have anti-proliferative, anti-neoplastic, anti-inflammatory, anti-epileptic, anti-ischemic, anti-diabetic, anti-psychotic, anti-nausea, anti-spasmodic, antibiotic, anti-anxiety, and anti-depressant functions. The anti-neoplastic action of cannabis—inhibiting development of malignant cells—was recognized in the 1970s and patented by the U.S. Department of Health and Human Services in 2003.[61]

If we simply look at the wording of the patents that the U.S. government has granted for cannabis, some of which are referenced in Chapter 2, we see some of these same medical terms describing its benefits as those used in Dr. Courtney's article, along with some new ones, such as analgesic, anti-emetic, sedative, anti-glaucoma, anti-tumoral, and neuroprotective activities. Remember, what's most important about any cannabis product are the qualities and attributes of the individual cannabinoids and other chemicals on their own, along with the entourage effect that comes from them collectively.

The book *Cannabis Chemotherapy* explains some of the ways through which cannabinoids and the human endocannabinoid system are believed to work together in treating cancer, as described in this excerpt:

The human endocannabinoid system and its plant-derived counterparts fight against cancer in a number of different ways, some of them utilizing mechanisms which are quite different from each other. One of the main mechanisms is the controlling of the process of natural programmed cell death (apoptosis) which causes a healthy cell to die when it is supposed to, instead of becoming a tumor.

A secondary function kicks in if a cell does become cancerous and continues to grow into a malignant tumor. Cannabinoids interrupt the signaling pathways that allow a growing malignant tumor to request that the body grow blood vessels to feed its growth. Interrupting this process, known as angiogenesis, simply causes the tumor to starve to death.

A third way that cannabinoids fight cancer is by directly attacking the cancer cells themselves, probably in much the same manner that traditional chemotherapy destroys them. But the difference is that cannabis does not harm the healthy cells surrounding the cancerous cells.

A fourth way that cannabinoids fight cancer is by providing nourishment to the human organism by stimulating the appetite. A well-fed human body has numerous mechanisms which kick in to fight for survival when under attack by disease of any kind. Preventing against starvation, due to greatly diminished appetite and aversion to food, is one of the most essential human survival responses. The creation of hunger utilizes mechanisms that are controlled by the endocannabinoid system and stimulated by plant-derived cannabinoids when necessary.[62]

The Ever-Evolving List of Conditions Being Treated with Cannabis

When you read the title of this chapter, "Every Patient's Question About Cannabis—Will It Help Me?" you may have expected a list of health conditions that have successfully been treated to follow. But if I were to include a list, it would be outdated before this book is published, since that list is constantly evolving. Also, if I included a list in this book and your condition wasn't on it, you might be discouraged and think that cannabis won't be helpful for you. When I first began my research on medical cannabis, I scoured books and websites, looking in vain for a reference to the condition I've been diagnosed with but there was very little out there. Over time, I finally found some references to patients who had found symptom relief with this condition and, I must say, knowing that some people with the same condition had been helped gave me a greater sense of hope that I would be helped too. That's a very human thing. Give me some evidence and I'll be soothed.

My feeling on the topic is this—if a condition exists that cannabis has not yet helped to one extent or another, I believe it will only be a matter of time until that happens. For that reason, searching for the specific health condition in books, videos and websites is your best bet for up-to-date research. In addition to determining that medical cannabis has helped patients with XYZ condition, if possible you'll also want to find as much information as possible about the specific cannabis strain(s) and/or the ratio of cannabinoids that have been effective for treating the condition.

Chapter 12

Is Cannabis Really a Safe Medicine?

It's important to understand and respect cannabis as the medicinal herb that it is. We need to use common sense and caution when we take it, just as we do with any other medicine. It's also important to honor the healing nature of the herb.

You are undoubtedly aware that many prescription and over-the counter medications contain warnings that you should not drive or use heavy machinery while you are taking them. Clearly, since even the smallest diminishment of your motor responses could lead to an accident, those warnings are there for a reason. It's no different if the medication is cannabis or a pharmaceutical painkiller, sleeping aid, or other drug that contains these warnings.

There are several different areas of safety to address on the subject of cannabis: questions about the product itself, concerns about overdosing, and the potential dangers of cannabis smoke.

Buying or Growing a Safe Cannabis Product

When the body is already dealing with compromised health, it's very important that everything you ingest is safe and free of any potential toxins. If you can obtain organically grown cannabis, that is preferred.

How do you know that a cannabis product is safe to use? While there is still a lot to do to be sure that medical marijuana is safe, it still trumps illegal or street cannabis, which may contain an extremely high ratio of THC, toxic additives, and/or synthetic ingredients. The sellers of street cannabis can offer absolutely no assurance to buyers that they are purchasing a safe product. But just because a cannabis product is sold as "legal" medical marijuana, that doesn't mean it is safe. The safety of medical cannabis depends on factors such as growing practices, quality control, and the use of professional manufacturing equipment.

In most cases, it's unlikely that we will ever know where a medical cannabis product was grown or how it was processed and handled. Therefore, it's imperative that we obtain it from sources that follow the highest of standards, including reproducible and reliable potency, composition, purity, and quality. Just as with the food, water, and beverages we consume, we expect those who sell medical cannabis to make safe products available. It is their responsibility to test samples of all batches of their products, preferably at high-quality independent labs. Testing for potency should verify the quantities of cannabinoids and other chemical compounds in the product. Safety testing should confirm that there are no residual solvents from the processing of cannabis products and no microbial contaminants, including pesticides, mold, spores, bacteria, viruses, insects, or parasites.

We need to be ever-diligent about the quality of any cannabis we take. Even if a product gives you relief from symptoms, that doesn't mean it's safe. There are recent reports on some products—in one case, they were high-CBD products—that caused patients to become "violently ill." It is very possible that these suspect products were grown on depleted soil that contained high levels of toxic metals and other contaminants or that they had undergone processing that involved toxic solvents.[63]

I visited the websites of several top cannabis testing labs and was pleased to see that a medical marijuana patient can obtain test results from them in a few days at a reasonable cost. However, be aware that some labs do not offer testing for toxic metals and other contaminants.

So what about growing your own? As I said earlier, the subject of growing cannabis is beyond the scope of this book; however, there are a number of websites and books on this topic if you are interested in growing your own. If you have the ability to do so and it is allowed by your state or jurisdiction, exploring the home-growing option might be a good choice. However, even if you have a green thumb and are extremely cautious, there's no guarantee that your plants will be free of mold, bacteria, or insect residue. For that reason, it's wise to have your home-grown cannabis lab-tested to determine the chemical profile and to confirm that it's safe.

Can a Person Overdose on Cannabis?

"Cannabis is the safest therapeutically-active substance on earth." That is a quote from a legal ruling by Francis L. Young, Administrative Law Judge at the U.S. Drug Enforcement Administration—yes, *the DEA*. By saying that cannabis is *the* safest therapeutically-active substance, it's clear to me that Judge Young understands how cannabis works and why it benefits the body in so many ways. Yet, as of this writing, Judge Young's 1988 decision that the federal government should allow medical use of cannabis is still not law. It was upheld by a Federal Appeals Court but then reversed on another appeal due to a technicality.[64]

Many of today's experts in medicine, science, law enforcement, and the judiciary agree with Judge Young's opinion, making one wonder how it is possible for cannabis to be considered *the safest* therapeutically-active substance we can find and yet, at the same time, condemned by many as a dangerous drug? Well, clearly, it's now obvious to more people that high-quality medical cannabis is *not* a dangerous drug; it is a healing herb. In all of my research, I have not found a single story about a death from overdosing on cannabis. That doesn't mean that cannabis doesn't pose addiction problems for some people; however, most experts who have studied the potential for cannabis addiction find that people who are addicted to or dependent upon cannabis in an unhealthy way may be psychologically addicted. But it's also NOT the dangerous drug that we've been brainwashed into believing it is for decades and decades. We'll go into further depth on the subject of addiction in the next chapter.

In the book, *Cannabis Chemotherapy*, David Hoye and his coauthors explain drug safety in the context of dosing and overdosing:

> Generally, drug safety is determined by the difference between the effective dose and the lethal dose. The greater the difference between the effective dose and the lethal dose, the safer the drug.
>
> The general measurement that scientists use to describe the difference is often referred to as the LD-50. LD stands for "lethal dose" and the figure of 50 refers to the dosage necessary to kill 50% of the lab mice in an experiment where all the mice were given equal amounts of the drug being tested. The LD-50 for cannabis has been determined to be extremely high. No human has ever died or even been injured by a cannabis overdose.

Although many adventurous cannabis users have used huge doses of oral cannabis to bring on trance and visions, some over and over on a regular basis, no one has ever died, or suffered physiological damage from these intense experiences. Emergency room doctors are well aware of this, and not all that infrequently get calls where someone has mistakenly eaten a confection which has been infused with cannabis medicine, or eaten a huge amount of cannabis edibles and are becoming worried because the effects are stronger than anticipated. The advice from the docs is always the same—sleep it off and you will be fine.[65]

What about the Dangers of Smoke?

When the question of safety comes up, another area that has caused concern is the smoke from cannabis joints. Since we know that cigarette smoking can lead to lung cancer, it's logical to assume that smoking isn't the safest or best way to use cannabis. But a government-sponsored study actually proved otherwise. Not only did the study disprove any connection between cannabis and lung cancer, it actually proved that *cannabis smokers who also smoke cigarettes gain a protective effect from the cannabis*. This is just one more arena in which the ubiquitous medicinal qualities of cannabis are down-right surprising. Here's how the authors of *Cannabis Chemotherapy* explain the study:

> In 2006 Dr. Donald Tashkin of UCLA released the results of his study on whether or not chronic, daily, long-term marijuana use causes lung cancer. ... this study was funded by the government in hopes that they could prove a scientific link between cannabis and lung cancer.

Dr. Tashkin was chosen as he had done many research studies for the government previously, most notably showing that the smoke from a joint of marijuana contains substantially higher concentrations of several classic cancer-causing chemicals than cigarettes. Because of these findings, Dr. Tashkin fully expected that his huge clinical study of thousands of daily smokers, over thirty years' time, would prove the obvious link. He believed, when embarking on this study, that it would prove that cannabis causes cancer.

Dr. Tashkin is an excellent scientist and an honest man. His study provided much proof regarding the link between lung cancer and pot smoking. But not in the way he, or the government, expected. His study showed that chronic long-term pot smoking does *not* cause an increase in lung cancer and, in fact, it actually protects against it! Even if a subject smokes cigarettes, his chances of developing cancer are lowered if he smokes cannabis also.

Dr. Tashkin honestly and unabashedly announced that long-term smoked cannabis has a protective effect against the very diseases that medical science thought it would cause. He was straightforward in admitting his surprise at the results of his study.

It is interesting to note that Dr. Tashkin has not been offered any funding for following up his study. He now speaks frequently at events at which the leading figures of the medical marijuana movement share their findings.[66]

Chapter 13

Will You Become Addicted to Medical Cannabis?

While medical cannabis has become much more accepted around the globe, it is likely that some people will think you are making a big mistake if you become a medical cannabis patient. They may have multiple concerns, but it's likely that addiction and psychoactivity will be among them. We'll address psychoactivity in greater detail in Chapter 14; meanwhile, let's explore the question of addiction.

When we ask the question, "Is medical cannabis addictive?" most studies confirm that only a small minority of cannabis users—nine percent according to most statistics—will become addicted to it. However, there is evidence that that statistic may be highly inflated—and some believe that any addictive aspect of cannabis is really a psychological addiction rather than a physical one, at least in most cases.

Comparing the Addiction Potential of Cannabis to Pharmaceutical Drugs

First, let's compare the addiction potential of cannabis to that of pharmaceutical drugs. A major television news channel host recently discussed the pros and cons of medical marijuana on his show. The host said that after a recent injury he was prescribed Vicodin, which gave him a high that was far beyond the high he ever got from his use of cannabis as a young man. That experience led him to question the logic behind Vicodin being given the status of a legally prescribed drug, while cannabis has been demonized by so many. Even the doctor he was interviewing, an addiction specialist who was vehemently opposed to medical marijuana, admitted that he has seen patients die from Vicodin, but knew of no deaths from marijuana. Yet, as of this writing, marijuana is still categorized by the U.S. government's Controlled Substances Act as a Schedule I drug—one of the most dangerous drugs available—while Vicodin is classified as a Schedule III drug, meaning that it supposedly has *less potential for abuse* than the drugs and other substances that are listed in Schedules I and II. Does that make any sense to you? If people have died from Vicodin but no deaths have ever been attributed to marijuana, which is the dangerous drug? Which one should be Schedule I and which should be Schedule III? Clearly, these designations are not scientifically accurate. When it comes to this natural medicine, governments, legislatures, and the public have been misguided by false information and scare tactics for many decades.

As I've mentioned, many addiction experts in the United States cite the often-stated statistic that nine percent of cannabis users are addicted to it. However, in *The Pot Book,* contributor Marsha Rosenbaum, PhD explains why she believes that statistic is so flawed. For decades, the "addict" label was attached to those who ended up in the criminal justice system for buying, using, or selling cannabis because, in many cases, the speediest path to get out of prison was to proclaim oneself an "addict," whether they were or not. Then, at a cost to those individuals and to society, they would be required to participate in a drug treatment program that they didn't need. Most were also labeled as an addict and a criminal for the rest of their lives.

Rosenbaum believes another factor that erroneously inflates the percentage of marijuana users who are "addicted" to nine percent is that many of those who are labeled as addicts have preexisting mental health problems. In these cases, Rosenbaum points out that it's likely that cannabis didn't *cause* the addiction; however the person's underlying mental condition could have led to an exacerbation of dependency on cannabis.[67]

Physical Addiction Versus Psychological Addiction

Some experts believe that the addictive potential of cannabis is mostly *psychological,* not *physical.* According to neuroscientist, psychiatrist, and brain imaging expert Dr. Daniel Amen, even when a physical addiction is caused by pharmaceutical and/or illegal drugs, there is also a psychological component involved. In other words, an addiction *can* be psychological only—or it can be *both* psychological and physical. In his book, *Unchain Your Brain*, Dr. Amen shares his finding that most people who struggle with addiction also hold the beliefs that they are bad, weak, or flawed.[68] He says addiction is a brain disease; it doesn't mean the addicted person is bad.

The emotional aspect of addiction is also addressed by Dr. Brené Brown in her book, *Daring Greatly: How the Courage to Be Vulnerable Transforms the Way We Live, Love, Parent, and Lead.* Dr. Brown suggests that the roots of addiction are "compulsive and chronic numbing of our feelings" and struggles with worthiness and shame, including feeling inadequate and "less than." She also cites anxiety and disconnection as factors, explaining that feelings of anxiety are fueled by uncertainty, overwhelming and competing demands on our time, and social discomfort; while *disconnection* includes a range of experiences, such as "depression, loneliness, isolation, disengagement, and emptiness."[69]

It's only when we *feel* the emotions that we've buried in our psyches that we're able to *heal* them. The emotional aspects of addiction are rooted in the many flawed premises—or to use Dr. Amen's term, ANTs or automatic negative thoughts—that constantly swim around inside our heads and keep us from much of the good that we want in life. It's human nature to struggle with this stuff. In the past, we learned to numb our feelings when that pit of loneliness and emptiness inside cried out for connection and worthiness. Now, it's time to heal those emotional woundings.

Let's look at the big picture on the issue of addiction—all addictions involve altered brain chemistry. Some people are addicted to compulsive behaviors such as gambling, video games, shopping, sex, or even running, while others are addicted to substances, including food, legal drugs, and illegal drugs.

When specific areas of the brain—referred to as its reward circuitry—are stimulated, the body produces pleasurable chemicals that make you feel good. Then, when you remember how good it felt, you have an inner urge to repeat the action that produced the feel-good chemicals so you can have that feeling again. And then your brain wants to feel it again—and again—and again. The pleasurable impact of the addictive substance or activity reinforces your desire for those specific substances or behaviors.

New research on the addiction potential of foods focused on a specific brand of cookie that's high in fat and sugar. The researchers found that people can become addicted to that cookie in the same way that they can become addicted to drugs. When this happens, they become tolerant to that specific brand of cookie and then, because of their increased tolerance level, they need to eat more and more cookies to get the pleasurable response. The body experiences such a strong desire for this specific food, and the high associated with it, that it becomes hyper-vigilant to cues that have become associated with this amazing cookie, just as if it were a drug they were addicted to.[70]

Now let's look at addiction to pharmaceutical drugs. One reason that people can become addicted to these drugs is that some of them are designed to mimic the body's own naturally-produced feel-good chemicals such as endorphins and dopamine. The problem is that when these chemicals are provided from an outside source, such as a drug, the body produces fewer of its own endorphins and dopamine. Even after only a short period of time, when a person decreases the amount of the drug they're taking or stops taking it altogether, there's a sudden drop in the amount of endorphins and dopamine in the body. Because the body has stopped producing as many of these feel-good chemicals itself—like it did before the person took the drug—it now has an insufficient amount to work with. Discontinuing the drug, especially if it's done suddenly, can lead to withdrawal symptoms such as anxiety, depression, insomnia, and chills—or, in rare instances, even life-threatening or fatal brain seizures.

When a drug interferes with the receptors in the brain in the ways I've described here, the potential for abuse is possible because the same mechanism that allows the drug to work in the way it was intended can lead to its misuse. There are numerous stories in the media of seemingly savvy, intelligent people who took drugs prescribed after an injury or an operation and then became hooked on them. In too many cases, an addiction to legal drugs leads to taking *illegal* drugs in short order, causing many honest, loving people to spiral downward, losing jobs, relationships, and a purpose for living. Some of them never recover from these addictions and, sadly, lose their lives.

When people become addicted, the body craves more and more of the desired drug. Those cravings can become so strong that it seems as though any intelligence they have flies out the window. Today there are dozens of potentially addictive pills on the market—and the disclaimers in their advertisements and television commercials are unnerving. More and more, we hear stories on the media about the negative effects of some of these drugs, such as people on sleep aids who were found sleep-walking and even "sleep-driving" in the middle of the night.

Once a person is addicted, the addiction cycle generally continues until—and *unless*—some type of intervention occurs. It can be self-intervention, intervention by family members, or intervention by the law. Before I began taking medical cannabis it was clear to me that I was, at the least, dependent on at least two of the three pharmaceutical drugs that I had been taking for some time. Occasionally, I wondered if I had already become a victim of unintentional, inadvertent addiction. As I mentioned earlier, just about every night I would awaken after a few hours and have to take an additional dose of one or more of the drugs in order to get a few more hours of sleep. I was taking *more* of the pills that both my doctor and I wanted to discontinue. I was feeling desperate because I knew about the potential for addiction and I certainly didn't want to become addicted to any of them. But sleep is such a precious commodity, and lack of sleep affects us mentally, emotionally, and physically. So it seemed that I was caught in a no-win situation. My body was crying out for a good night's rest but, despite the pharmaceutical drugs, I didn't sleep well. This happens to lots of patients. A medical doctor told me that she'd also become hooked on the same prescription sleeping pill that I took—and the only way she was finally able to get off it was to go cold turkey. But it was a very challenging process for her. She was up all day and all night, totally unable to sleep, for five days. Then, finally, her exhausted body went to sleep and she was no longer addicted to the pill.

Thankfully, medical cannabis has allowed me to sleep better than I have in years—and it's also provided other amazing beneficial effects for me. How do I know that I'm not addicted? On a few occasions over the past couple of years, I forgot to take it at bedtime. Lying in bed, drifting off to sleep, the realization that I hadn't taken my cannabis medicine would come to my mind. Sometimes, I got up and took it. But on a few evenings, I was so close to sleep that I drifted off without doing so. On those nights, I didn't have the pain relief that cannabis provides and therefore didn't sleep as well as usual. The next morning, I definitely felt more tired than usual. But the big insight from this experience—and the reason I'm sharing it with you—is that I *did* sleep those nights. I didn't sleep as well without the cannabis, but I *did* sleep.

A New Perspective on Addiction and the Brain

In his bestselling book, *The Brain's Way of Healing,* psychiatrist and psychoanalyst Norman Doidge, MD, describes his own research, as well as that of other pioneers in the new field of science and medicine, *neuroplasticity.* Neuroplasticity is the understanding that the brain is "plastic" and highly dynamic—and that mental abilities that have been lost due to damage or disease can be recovered by using the brain's own inherent sophistication to achieve that healing. This is a major shift in the understanding of the way the brain works. In essence, neuroplasticity allows us to "rewire' the brain through natural, noninvasive avenues.

Dr. Doidge's book includes a chapter on the amazing findings of Michael H. Moskowitz, MD, a psychiatrist and pain medicine specialist. Dr. Moskowitz suffered two different life-threatening accidents that caused severe injuries and pain. The pain was so excruciating that, many days, he was unable to work. As a pain specialist who was facing his own battle with ongoing chronic pain, Dr. Moskowitz realized that the only treatments that were available to him and his patients were almost totally ineffective for the level of pain experienced by many. Morphine and other painkillers, anti-inflammatory drugs, physical therapy, traction, massage, self-hypnosis, rest, ice, heat—these treatments barely touched the pain he was dealing with all day, every day. After thirteen years of dealing with pain, it was getting more severe, not better.

Dr. Doidge also writes about Dr. Moskowitz's insights on how quickly drugs like opioids can become addictive:

> One of Moskowitz's most important insights is that the new opioid narcotics, so popular for pain treatment, have actually made many pain problems worse, because neither the drug companies nor many physicians take into account the role of neuroplasticity in pain. Opioid narcotics, the most potent pain medications we have, generally don't work well over long periods of time. Often within days or weeks, patients become "tolerant" to such a drug; the size of the initial dose loses its effect, so they need ever more medication, or they experience "breakthrough pain" while on the drug. But as the dose is increased, so too is the danger of addiction and overdose. To better block pain, drug companies invented "long-acting" opioids, such as OxyContin, a long-acting morphine. People with chronic pain would often be placed on OxyContin-like drugs for life.
>
> As we've seen, the brain makes its own opioidlike substances to block pain, and the manufactured drugs supplement them by attaching to the brain's own opioid receptors. As long as scientists believed that the brain couldn't change, they never anticipated that bombarding the opioid receptors with opioid medications could do harm. However, says Moskowitz, "once we saturate all our God-given receptors, the brain produces new ones." It adapts to being inundated by long-term opioids by becoming less sensitive to them—and thus patients become more sensitive to pain, and more dependent on their drugs, which can make their chronic pain worse. The problem exists, says Moskowitz, with all the pain medicines.

Once he made his discoveries, he slowly began to wean many patients from their long-term opioids. A key to success was to lower the dose very slowly, thereby giving the neuroplastic brain the time it needed to adapt to being without drugs, so the patient wouldn't experience any "breakthrough pain." Tapering slowly, down to 50 to 80 percent of the original dose, could break the cycle of opioid pain sensitivity.[71]

In comparing the addiction potential of cannabis with pharmaceutical drugs, the authors of *Cannabis Chemotherapy* explain:

> The definition of addiction that usually accompanies drug use issues is based around what happens when one stops using a drug that has been consumed regularly over an extended period of time. Synthetic and organic opioids, OxyContin, heroin, Vicodin, etc., produce severe withdrawal symptoms when extended use is ended abruptly. These usually consist of vomiting, extreme overall body pain, extreme depression, overall flu-like symptoms, alternating periods of sweats and shivers, etc. Strangely, these are quite similar to the regular side effects of traditional chemotherapy in those who tolerate it poorly.
>
> When cannabis use, even chronic long-term daily cannabis use, is abruptly ended, one might undergo slight bouts of nervousness, restlessness, and a change in sleep patterns. These symptoms subside and disappear after just a few days.
>
> In those who found the so-called side effects to be pleasurable, there may be a desire to keep experiencing the side effects once the body has rid itself of cancer. Because science indicates that continued use of cannabis may prevent or lower the chances of relapse, and because there are no

known negative physical repercussions, continued cannabis use may be a favored option by any cancer survivor. And while some with inflexible anti-drug warrior mindsets might look at this as an addiction, those with common sense will likely see it as a continuing cancer prevention therapy.[72]

Chapter 14

What About Potential Side Effects and Psychoactivity?

We've looked at the many beneficial effects of cannabis medicine; now let's focus on the "side effects"—the feelings and physical experiences in the bodies and minds of patients. In this chapter, we'll also look at the detoxing and psychoactive aspects of the herb in greater detail, including more about the types of products that cause little or no psychoactivity.

Possible Side Effects from Cannabis

Below I've listed some of the more common side effects that people experience from cannabis.

- Mood enhancement
- Euphoria
- Deep relaxation
- Sedative effect
- Reduced anxiety *or* increased anxiety
- Enhanced awareness of one's surroundings
- Heightened sense of well-being

- Altered sense of time and space
- Heightened creativity
- Hunger, also known as the munchies
- Weight loss (for those who need to lose weight)
- Uncontrollable laughter or giddiness
- Heightened sense of taste and/or smell
- Decrease in short-term memory
- Disorganized thinking

Some of these side effects, such as the first one listed, "mood enhancement," should be positive for all patients; while others may be positive for some and negative for others. In fact, two different patients who are taking the exact same strain and dose of cannabis may have opposite experiences.

Uncomfortable side effects, such as increased anxiety, decrease in short-term memory, or disorganized thinking may result from overdosing. Or, a person who takes too much cannabis might suddenly feel so relaxed that they are very tired. That's okay if it's bedtime but if you have a full day ahead of you, it could be problematic. And a possible cause of increased anxiety could be the long-time illegal status of cannabis. I understand that; I've never been in prison but even the thought of that possibility definitely produces anxiety.

Then there's the stereotype that many people associate with cannabis—you'll get the munchies and gain weight. Thankfully, no munchies for me. In fact, I have lost weight using cannabis, which was a good thing for me, and probably due to the homeostasis it provides to the body. However, for patients who are suffering from nausea, the munchies are a great gift. You see, the old stereotypes don't apply to all people or all strains of cannabis, especially many of the strains used for *medicinal* purposes. People who need to lose weight often do, while many people who need to gain weight find that their appetite improves.

Detoxing as Part of the Healing Process

Holistic doctors, including homeopaths, naturopaths, osteopaths, chiropractors, and acupuncturists often explain to their patients that true healing usually involves the release of toxins from the body, and an uncomfortable side effect of that process is that we sometimes feel sicker for a while before we begin to feel better. This detoxing process, which some doctors refer to as an *aggravation* or a *healing crisis*, occurs when the cells detox faster than the body can keep up.

When I first started taking cannabis medicine, I would occasionally burp or feel a brief flutter of mild nausea that would give me a minute or two of slight discomfort and then pass. Even though these symptoms didn't feel "good," detoxing is exactly what I want so I consider any mild symptoms as a positive sign. However, sometimes detox symptoms are more challenging, such as extreme tiredness, nausea, fever, a runny nose, diarrhea, or loss of appetite. If they are too challenging to deal with, fine-tuning the dose might help to minimize those effects, while still leading you in the direction of symptom relief and healing. Of course, if the symptoms concern you, check with your health practitioner.

Bruce Fife, ND, is a leading edge holistic doctor whose book, *The Healing Crisis*, explains what usually happens when the body is in a cleansing mode:

> The healing crisis is an inherent part of the healing process. Sometimes the crisis is severe as heavy cleansing occurs. At other times the crisis may be all but unnoticeable as cleansing may be operating at a slower pace. But cleansing is occurring—it must occur in order to bring about renewed health. ...
>
> Contrary to popular belief, exposure to germs is not the reason people get colds. Bacteria, viruses, fungi, and other pathogenic organisms are constantly in and on our bodies.

They are everywhere, and everybody is exposed to them. For example, the rhinovirus, which causes the common cold, is always present, but we don't all have colds because it is kept under control by our immune system. Rhinovirus can only proliferate and cause problems when the immune system becomes weakened by a toxic overload, by physical or mental stress, or other negative factors. It is a well-established fact that cold temperatures do not cause colds, nor does exposure to other sick people. Colds are passed around only among those people who have weak immune systems. Healthy people with strong immune systems can come in contact with those who have highly contagious diseases without "catching" their illness.

... Sickness is, in effect, a cleansing process. If the body has the strength and nutrients it needs, then the illness is overcome and the body regains health. Because of the cleansing, we may be healthier immediately after the sickness than before. A condition that causes the body to expel toxins is referred to as a cleansing crisis. ...

If the body is too weak or adequate nourishment is not provided to fight off the invading germs and cleanse toxic substances, the illness will be prolonged. Nutrients vital to good health may be used up in the process and, if not quickly replenished, the deficiency will lead to some degree of malnutrition and all of its accompanying consequences. The person will still feel sick even after the major symptoms have subsided. These are the type of individuals who are at greatest risk from potentially deadly viruses and bacterial infections.

...When we become sick, our body is telling us to rest so it can focus its healing energies on housecleaning (detoxification). Symptoms of sickness—runny nose, fever, diarrhea, nausea, sneezing, coughing, loss of appetite, etc.—are all processes of cleansing.[73]

As a patient increases or decreases his dosage or switches to a different cannabis product to achieve the greatest efficacy possible, additional detoxing symptoms may occur. Detoxing is a natural process but it can be a bit disconcerting when you are *finally* starting to feel better again and then dip into the frustration of *more* discomfort in the body. But it is so important to let the body heal according to its own needs—and detoxing is not a bad thing; actually, it is our goal.

Dealing with the Psychoactive Effects

Now let's look at psychoactivity. The experience of the high or stoned feeling from cannabis is caused by the activated THC, which acts in the brain's reward system by stimulating brain cells to release the chemical dopamine. The high can vary considerably from one person to the next—ranging from minor, almost indistinguishable effects to more obvious changes in sensory perceptions, mood, cognition, and behavior. It can result in pleasant feelings or negative feelings, as well as increased alertness or heightened senses.

While most people can deal with *some* psychoactivity—and many people enjoy the high or stoned feeling—there are patients who do not tolerate its effects very well. I am one of them. Because my balance and coordination are already impaired to a degree—and because I am highly sensitive to THC—its psychoactive quality makes me even more wobbly. When I take cannabis with more than a smidgen of THC, it sometimes doesn't even feel safe to take a trip to the bathroom in the middle of the night. On numerous occasions I made the attempt but was unsuccessful—putting one foot on the floor, putting some weight on it with a bit of uncertainty, and then giving up when my attempt to put the other foot on the floor made it clear that it might not go well. On those occasions, I would tell my bladder that it had no choice but to hold on for a couple of hours. These experiences made me realize that having a cane near my bed was an imperative in the event of any nighttime emergencies. So I appropriated a pedestal cane—the type with three or four little "feet" at the bottom—from the back of a closet, since that type of cane provides more stability.

A majority of those who are opposed to the use of marijuana believe that this psychoactive high or stoned reaction is reason enough to block its legalization for all of us. Most of them seem to be taking an anti-marijuana stance because of the effects of this one chemical. They don't seem to understand that **NOT all** forms of cannabis are high in THC—and that some of the newer medicinal strains of cannabis are actually **LOW** in THC.

To say it another way, these anti-marijuana adherents are basing their stance on the flawed idea that all marijuana is basically the same. While it's true that most of the back-alley cannabis strains that have influenced the thinking of anti-marijuana adherents contain an extremely high ratio of THC, and therefore cause a lot of psychoactivity for many users, not all strains of cannabis cause that degree of psychoactivity and some strains and forms cause little to no psychoactivity. Based on studies of medical literature from the late 1800s and early 1900s, many of today's experts believe that the strains of cannabis used then contained much, much lower ratios of THC and were much higher in CBD and other cannabinoids that are considered to be more healing in nature.

Some experts believe that CBD may reduce the level of psychoactivity caused by THC. They credit the entourage effect—the way in which the chemicals work together in the body—to explain why some people experience reduced psychoactivity when a cannabis product contains substantial amounts of *both* THC and CBD. In other words, the CBD counteracts the effects of the THC, lessening or, in some cases, almost eliminating its psychoactive qualities.[74]

Strains of cannabis in the categories of nutritional or industrial hemp also have a very low amount of THC and therefore should not cause any psychoactivity. Because they do *not* fall under marijuana laws, these strains can be sold without restriction in Canada and Europe, with THC content limited to under 0.3 percent in Canada and under 1 percent in Europe. As of this writing, other jurisdictions seem to be more lenient toward nutritional and industrial hemp, but they make it confusing since they skirt the issue of what's legal and what's not. Many nutritional and industrial hemp products are now being marketed—and some medical marijuana products also fall into this category due to their very low THC content.

Another consideration about psychoactivity that many who hold strong anti-marijuana stances may not understand is that they themselves are probably using substances that cause psychoactive effects. *Any food or substance that alters brain function and causes changes in perception, mood, or behavior is considered to be psychoactive.* That includes coffee and chocolate, both of which contain caffeine, as well as alcohol and tobacco. Anyone who uses any of these foods or substances is experiencing psychoactivity to some degree. All you need to do is focus on how you feel after you have imbibed coffee, chocolate, alcohol, or tobacco. The difference in mood may be subtle, but for most individuals it's still distinguishable when you really tune in to how your body and your mind feel.

While it may be easy to dismiss the psychoactive effects of some foods and substances which many of us use on a daily basis, a number of pharmaceutical drugs—both over-the-counter and prescription—cause psychoactivity to a degree that is much more significant than some realize. Some over the counter drugs, such as cough and cold remedies that contain dextromethorphan, can cause hallucinations when taken in excess. And as we reviewed in Chapter 13, many common prescription drugs also bring with them the possibility of addictive and psychoactive qualities. They include narcotics that are used for pain management, stimulants used to treat narcolepsy and attention disorders, and antidepressants and antipsychotics that are used to treat neurological and psychiatric conditions.

In Chapter 20, you will learn about three different categories of cannabis products that, in almost all cases, do not produce a psychoactive high. I believe that all patients should be able to access a range of cannabis products since we know that very different ratios of THC, CBD, and other cannabinoids are efficacious for different health conditions. While I'm thrilled that more high-CBD products are now becoming available, we don't want to throw THC out with the bathwater. For some conditions, cannabis that includes a quantity of THC will be the most efficacious, with studies showing that this specific chemical can be helpful for pain relief (especially neuropathic pain), post traumatic stress disorder, nausea, vomiting, asthma, glaucoma, insomnia, and as an appetite stimulant.

When it comes to the high or stoned experience, cannabis doesn't cause it to be pleasant *or* negative; it simply amplifies the energy that you're already expressing in your consciousness. It might bring with it the attributes of a stimulant, a depressant, or a hallucinogen. On the negative end of the spectrum, some medical cannabis patients experience hallucinations, paranoia, anxiety, or impaired motor skills that could cause dizziness and lead to an accident. If one takes too much, nausea and vomiting could result or, in an extreme situation, a patient might even experience chest pains.

Each individual experiences the psychoactive nature of cannabis in their own unique way. Although potency and dosage are obvious factors, some people have developed a tolerance to THC, saying that high-THC cannabis doesn't make them high at all. Also, sometimes the results an individual experiences vary from one day to the next, even when taking the same product in the same dosage. A lack of psychoactive effects could be due to the subtleties of the sensation a person is experiencing, or it's possible that the amount a person took was too small to produce any noticeable effects.

Some of the "trips" that cannabis has taken me on have bordered on scary, some were just plain weird, some were fun, and others were beautiful. Oftentimes, a single "trip" has included all of those experiences—with a fun experience fading into a scary scene or a weird experiencing morphing into something beautiful.

To the extent that the "trip" is an inevitable part of the cannabis experience, I have learned to maximize it, as I'll explain shortly. Many people say that it leads to greater creativity and problem-solving abilities. One friend tells me that she thinks of this time as a mini-vacation during which she mentally steps into a change of pace that includes deep relaxation and the ability to leave her usual thoughts and concerns behind.

So why does cannabis have psychoactive qualities anyway? As I shared earlier, the "trip" that is enticing and desirable to so many is something I prefer to avoid because it causes me to be more wobbly. Since my health challenge already makes me wobbly, it comes down to a safety issue for me. However, I suspect that I would feel the same way about the high even if I didn't have the issue with wobbliness. Perhaps that's because I like to be in control and it feels as if the high is something that my conscious mind can't totally control. Those experiences made me wonder if cannabis makes us high because Nature wants to distract us, giving us a much-needed break from the ongoing chatter of self-talk in our minds, much of which is focused on negative issues or worries.

Recent findings on the healing effects of the high, including the ways cannabis can heal us psychologically from conditions such as post traumatic stress disorder (PTSD), are addressed in an article entitled *Worth Repeating: Marijuana and the Psychology of Optimal Experience*. Here is an excerpt:

> As counterintuitive as it sounds, the "high" or "feel good" buzz from marijuana is an actual "therapeutic effect" that heals the

brain, produces homeostasis and prevents many neurodegenerative conditions.

Brain homeostasis is restored by the direct action of THC/CBD-activating CB1 receptors in the amygdala which regulate our "happiness/emotional salience module." This pathway is dedicated to seeking for "meaningfulness" in our existence.

This innate drive is the need for self-actualization. THC increases the probability of these events occurring, through inducing metaphysical "flow states" and "peak experiences." We live near the edge, where the view is better.

This plant, with its deep historical partnership with the human species, continues to amaze medical researchers who now are trying to decipher the workings of the endocannabinoid system. The latest research evidence is now concluding that the cannabinoid system, when activated, helps the amygdala unlearn the response people may experience from past major fearful events that keep returning ... as the latest research from the Max Planck Institute of Psychiatry/Research Group Neuronal Plasticity (Germany's Harvard) is reporting.

Imagine that! Medical marijuana helps the brain unlearn fear! [Emphasis mine] One might describe marijuana's effects as producing flow, as the opposite of "amygdala hijack," as seen in PTSD. Marijuana resets a damaged amygdala which is in a hyper-alert fear state.

The amygdala performs primary roles in the formation and storage of memories associated with emotional events. Research indicates that, during fear conditioning, sensory stimuli reach the basolateral complexes of the amygdala, particularly the lateral nuclei, where they form associations with memories of the stimuli. The association between stimuli and the aversive events they predict may be mediated by long-term potentiating, a sustained enhancement of signaling between affected neurons. Additionally, data demonstrate that acute marijuana smoking produced minimal effects on complex cognitive task performance in experienced marijuana users.

Marijuana's effects are humanistic; they support human wellness in body and mind. The psychological states of flow, peak experience, and self-actualization experiences are generated by cannabis use and using medical, whole-plant marijuana and getting "high" is good for you, for your cognitive and emotional health.

Or as lifelong marijuana user, Dr. Carl Sagan, an exemplar of self-actualization, said: "I am convinced that there are genuine and valid levels of perception available with cannabis (and probably with other drugs) which are, through the defects of our society and our educational system, unavailable to us without such drugs. The illegality of cannabis is outrageous, an impediment to full utilization of a drug which helps produce the serenity and insight, sensitivity and fellowship so desperately needed in this increasingly mad and dangerous world." Carl Sagan, in Dr. Lester Grinspoon's *Marijuana Reconsidered.*

Medical marijuana is positive psychology psychotherapy in plant-based form.[75]

I love the last sentence in this article so much that I'm going to repeat it: "Medical marijuana is *positive psychology psychotherapy* in plant-based form [Emphasis mine]." Science is now backing up a concept that many recreational users of cannabis have hyped for years—their belief that cannabis expands their consciousness in a positive way. The idea that cannabis helps us to heal psychological wounds by "unlearning fears" that are rooted in the amygdala of the brain might also explain a bit about why it is also such a great mood-enhancer.

An Israeli medical cannabis study showed overall improvement for 19 nursing home residents, as detailed in an article on the website http://ScienceDaily.com. Here's an excerpt:

> ... 19 patients between the ages of 69 and 101 were treated with medical cannabis in the form of powder, oil, vapor, or smoke three times daily over the course of a year for conditions such as pain, lack of appetite, and muscle spasms and tremors. Researchers and nursing home staff monitored participants for signs of improvement, as well as improvement in overall life quality, such as mood and ease in completing daily living activities.
>
> During the study, 17 patients achieved a healthy weight, gaining or losing pounds as needed. Muscle spasms, stiffness, tremors and pain reduced significantly. Almost all patients reported an increase in sleeping hours and a decrease in nightmares and PTSD-related flashbacks.
>
> There was a notable decline in the amount of prescribed medications taken by patients, such as antipsychotics, Parkinson's treatment, mood stabilizers, and pain relievers, Klein found, noting that these drugs have severe side effects. By the end of the study, 72 percent of participants were able to reduce their drug intake by an average of 1.7 medications a day.[76]

It's a pretty good bet that all of the patients in that study received exactly the same cannabis products. That makes sense in terms of a controlled study; however, it would be fascinating if each of those patients got a strain of cannabis that was specifically chosen for their needs. I see the day coming when cannabis medicine is much more targeted so each individual can achieve maximum benefit.

Directing the Trajectory of My "Trips"

Over time, even though I didn't seem to be able to stop the "trip" that cannabis took me on, I realized that I could learn to focus what was going on in my head during the "trip" and then consciously direct it. When a person's trip is on a negative trajectory, it's not the cannabis that is causing the negative experience. The trip simply amplifies the emotional set-point that is active in the person's consciousness.

In her book, *The Yoga of Marijuana*, Joan Bello explains that the reaction we experience on the trip is correlated to the emotional set-point that is active in our consciousness:

> The extent and depth of our hidden demons determines the degree of the paranoid reaction that may erupt. Nevertheless, to face our bare selves is a necessary, if sometimes painful but ultimately rewarding development. Luckily, regular jaunts into reality implemented via Marijuana allow for growth in self-knowledge without the initial shock that can cause the short-lived distress.[77]

At some point in time, I realized that I didn't have to just let a scene in my head play out in the direction it was currently going. Instead, when I *focused* on what was happening in the scene and then made a conscious decision to create a different scene, I found that I could easily and quickly do that. In some respects, this ability to direct the way the scene is unfolding is similar to lucid dreaming, in which the dreamer becomes aware *during the dream* that he is dreaming. If you've ever experienced a lucid dream, when you became aware that you were in the middle of a dream you were probably surprised—*and, at the same time, you also knew that you could influence and change the direction of the dream or what was happening in the dream.* My experience with a cannabis trip is very similar to this.

I learned that whether the trip was pleasant or negative, I was able to direct it. The big distinction between the two types of trips is that I had no reason or desire to change the focus or scene of the pleasant trips. But when I found myself on a negative trip, I learned that I could make a conscious decision and change what was going on in my head. This didn't always happen right away because sometimes it was as if I *forgot* that I could rewrite the scene that was playing out in my head. Curled up in bed and feeling the relaxation that the cannabis induced in my body, it sometimes took a bit of time for me to realize it when I was focused on a negative scene. Then I would have to take charge, saying to myself, "Wait a minute, I don't like this scene. I'm going to change the scene I'm seeing in my head to something I like better." But, first, I had to focus on what I wanted that new scene to be. Then, just as if I switched to a different TV channel, a totally different scene would unfold in my "head trip." What an analogy for my life! When I get focused on something negative, it *always* feels better when I make a conscious decision that I want to feel better. But I have to *want* to do that, which sometimes involves making a conscious decision to turn my thoughts away from something that's troubling me and soothe myself as I align with something more positive.

I eventually learned that it only took a little bit of focus and effort for me to consciously take control of—or direct—my cannabis trips. To me, any time we consciously choose to feel better emotionally, we are stepping into an opportunity for a happier life. But—and this is a big BUT—we have to *want* to feel better.

As discussed in Chapter 10, we've all experienced emotional woundings in our lives that are the direct result of flawed premises we hold. These woundings wouldn't have happened in the first place if we didn't believe untruths about our innate nature and our innate value. Subconscious beliefs such as "I'm *less than* others," or "I never get a break in life," or "I'm not smart enough" keep us trapped in mediocrity, victim consciousness, fear, powerlessness, and depression. When we consciously identify the negative or limiting thoughts in our everyday lives and then consciously make the decision to shift our focus to a positive thought or image instead, we are learning to focus our consciousness and direct our thoughts in positive directions.

When I finally connected the dots, I realized that when I refocus the direction of a less-than-desirable cannabis trip in order to shift it in a positive direction, I am actually doing the exact same thing that I do in my everyday life. That's because, for some years now, I have been—bit by bit—letting go of the sloppy, lazy thinking that can quickly take my mind off into negative directions. More and more, I find that I am able to "catch" a limited or negative thought as it's rolling along in my head and shift it to a positive mode by finding a better-feeling thought on the subject at hand.

Once again, I turn to marijuana researcher Joan Bello, whose insights in *The Benefits of Marijuana* help to explain how cannabis calms the brain and positively impacts its functioning:

> When the system is hyper-aroused, as in today's lifestyle, marijuana calms. The significance of this fact cannot be ignored. It explains the increased creativity reported as a part of the marijuana experience, because when both sides of brain processes are heightened, both types of brain activity are greater. The left brain notices more, while the right brain receives more. This is the unification of logic and intuition. The term "expansion of consciousness" is explained physiologically as a "shifting of brain emphasis from one-sidedness to balance" (Sugarman and Tarter, 1978), which fits precisely with the feeling called "high."
>
> Marijuana ingestion has been shown to change the worried state by producing alpha waves, experienced as well being.

When we ingest marijuana, the heart swells through capillary enhancement and is fueled more by more fully oxygenated blood, while, at the same time, its contractions and expansions are greater, allowing for stronger pumping action to the rest of the body.

As rigidity in the body is released or reduced by the action of marijuana, there is a corresponding reduction of mental tension that translates into a feeling of expansion and wellbeing and explains the reverential attitude commonly expressed by marijuana lovers.

As the body's workings can become more harmonious with marijuana, the functioning of the five senses can be noticeably improved. ... In our discussion, the trigger to the high experience is marijuana, but many other activities can also produce it, such as jogging, chanting, fasting, isolation, meditation, and prayer.[78]

The experiences of the psychoactive high can vary greatly from one patient to another—and those experiences can range from very mild to extremely intense. For most patients, the high from the THC in cannabis diminishes over time as their tolerance increases. That's why patients who are taking a high-THC cannabis product are generally told to start with a very small dose and increase it gradually if a higher dose is desirable. But some medical cannabis patients can tolerate only a small amount of psychoactivity; in some cases, none at all. As I mentioned earlier, I'm one of those patients for whom psychoactivity is undesirable. When I take a cannabis product that causes psychoactivity, I generally do so before bed at night, because THC makes me wobbly. Unlike most people, whose bodies create a tolerance to THC, my body has achieved only a minimal amount of tolerance even though I've now been taking it for a couple of years.

Another variable with cannabis is that two people might experience the same "effect," but interpret it in totally different ways.

For one person, a specific side effect might be "positive," while another person might label a similar experience as "negative." Why is it possible for two people to have such a range of experiences from the exact same substance? In addition to the differences in body chemistry and other aspects of their physiology, there is a great deal of scientific evidence that your beliefs will impact your experience. Again, when we look at research on the placebo effect, it is clear that *your expectations* of positive or negative side effects from medical cannabis—or any other medication or treatment—may be responsible, or partly responsible, for those positive or negative effects *in your body*.

I now see the experience of the high as a gift from the Universe that has allowed me to achieve a greater ability to focus and greater emotional healing, rather than as a bothersome effect.

Chapter 15

How to Talk to Your Doctor about Cannabis Medicine

IMPORTANT NOTE

Now that some companies are selling high-CBD, low-THC cannabis products under the category of "nutritional supplements," it's possible that you may NOT need a doctor's recommendation to get a strain and form of cannabis that will help you. However, every patient's needs are different. Some conditions require a much higher quantity of THC than is available in high-CBD, low-THC products. Patients for whom that is the case may experience more efficacy with a cannabis medicine that falls under medical marijuana laws. Also, as of this writing, the legality of these "very low THC" products is a gray area.

Picture this: On a regular visit with your doctor, she brings up the subject of medical cannabis and explains why it might be helpful for your health condition(s). She gives you a prescription or whatever other paperwork is necessary where you live and also reviews with you all of the possibilities of the strain, type, form, and potency of cannabis medicine that might be best for your needs.

Wouldn't it be great if your own personal doctor was knowledgeable about medical cannabis and able to guide you through the process of using it in the most beneficial way? Though it may be a while before the average physician will be as progressive about medical cannabis as you might like, don't simply assume that your physician isn't up for the discussion. It's possible that it may be easier than you think to discuss the possibilities with her and she may surprise you and turn into your best ally on the subject. So I suggest giving her at least one chance to be the progressive doctor you want her to be.

With all of the media reports on the many different health conditions that cannabis has eased or healed, more doctors are waking up to its life-giving properties. If your doctor is already well-versed in integrative medicine, holistic health, or herbal medicine, she may be extremely receptive. Of course, even the most savvy alternative practitioner probably wouldn't go so far as suggesting that you break the law to use cannabis, so if you live in a jurisdiction that *doesn't* yet legally allow medical marijuana or "recreational" marijuana, talk to her about the new "legal everywhere" high-CBD options that can even be ordered on the Internet.

Even if you believe that your own doctor would be the *last* doctor on earth to recommend that you take cannabis, don't just assume that she will have a negative reaction to it. Having said that, I don't know your doctor—and I do acknowledge that there are some doctors who probably won't budge on this topic. So, if it truly feels like your doctor is stuck in the limited world of allopathic medicine, I understand that you may decide to pass on having that conversation. And that's okay too, because you can pursue other options.

If you live in a jurisdiction where medical marijuana is legal, that means your government honors the medicinal value of cannabis. And that means you have every right to discuss this medication with your doctor. However, in most jurisdictions where it is legal there is a lot of red tape that a doctor must deal with to legally recommend cannabis and many doctors don't have the time or inclination to deal with all of the regulations.

As I shared earlier, my doctor agreed that medical cannabis might be helpful for me and referred me to another doctor, from whom I got the required state "recommendation" that made me a legal medical marijuana patient. His nearby clinic was modern and clean; nowhere did I see any reference to cannabis. It was a "real" medical clinic, not a fly-by-night clinic that might disappear in short order like some I had heard about. I completed some paperwork and then, after a short wait, a nurse took my blood pressure and weight, and asked me some questions. Then the doctor came in, reviewed my file, asked me some more questions, gave me a brief exam, and told me the nurse would give me the paperwork I needed to obtain medical cannabis.

I was relieved that it was all so simple and easy. No icky back alleys, scary characters lurking around, or dirty clinics. I hope you'll check the reputation of any doctor you're thinking of seeing, which is important for a couple of reasons. Obviously, you want a doctor you can trust. And you want to be sure the doctor who prepares your paperwork is going to be around awhile. Depending on your local laws, you may need a renewal after a certain period of time and starting over with a new doctor would take more time and probably cost more money. Also, if there is ever a legal challenge to your use of cannabis, you want to be sure that your paperwork came from a bona fide physician with the legal right to "prescribe" cannabis. Hopefully this type of legal challenge will be happening less and less in the future, but if it happens to you, having a reputable doctor's name on your paperwork—a doctor whose medical opinion is not suspect— could be helpful.

If you live in a jurisdiction where medical cannabis is legal, there are lots of options for finding a doctor who will provide you with the needed paperwork. If you have supportive friends or relatives, ask if they know of a doctor who can recommend marijuana—or go to nearby marijuana stores and ask there. Another option is to do a web search for doctors in your area by searching "medical marijuana doctor" and including your city's name or your zip code in the search so the results will provide local information. When you make an appointment, be sure to find out what medical records they need you to take with you, including test results and any prescriptions you are currently taking.

Next, we'll look at where you can get medical cannabis.

Chapter 16

Where to Get Your Cannabis Medicine—And Should You Grow It?

Today, more medical cannabis products are available than ever before, giving patients numerous choices that range in strain type, form, and potency. But how do you know where to go, what to buy, whose suggestions to trust, or what to expect? And is it possible for you to grow your own?

Finding a Medical Cannabis Store Near You

In my part of the world there are stores nearby that prominently display signs with a large green cross, signifying that they are licensed to sell medical cannabis. But I didn't like the idea of just walking into one and buying whatever a sales clerk recommended.

When I first pursued cannabis as a medicine, the only solid upfront guidance that I had about my choices was from a knowledgeable friend who told me about a specific cannabis product that had been efficacious for a friend of hers. Since I didn't want to smoke cannabis, I was really glad to hear that this product came in capsule form.

I wanted to be sure that I could get the brand of cannabis capsules that were effective for my friend's friend, so I went to the store she told me about, even though it was a 30-minute drive. I didn't mind the drive because I knew they carried the product she recommended. And I was really glad I made that decision because when I later decided to visit a couple of nearby marijuana stores to see what they carried, I learned that neither of them carried any products in capsule form. I had assumed that every marijuana store sold some type of capsule but, at least at that point in time, I was wrong about that. I learned that all marijuana stores DON'T sell the same items so, if you don't find what you want, go elsewhere.

If you live in an area that gives you multiple options for purchasing medical cannabis, I suggest that you check out at least a few of them so you'll know the types of products that are available. In my state, marijuana stores are called dispensaries or collectives; some are small and cramped, while others are larger and look more like a variation on a pharmacy. Some stores carry dozens of different types of cannabis products while, at others, cannabis is available mostly in more traditional forms for smoking, vaporizing, etc.

Charities and Online Cannabis Retailers

Some medical cannabis charities supply cannabis to patients at a discount or even for free. How do you find out about them? I suggest that you do research online and also ask anyone who might have anything to do with medical cannabis if they know of any charity that helps patients.

As of this writing, the only companies that sell medical cannabis online across state lines are those that are high in CBD and extremely low in THC strains, which I refer to as "legal everywhere."

Finding the Right Cannabis Medicine for You

While the media continues to report about new strains of cannabis that are helping patients with very specific health challenges, at this point in time most patients are still not able to purchase cannabis medicine that is targeted for their own unique needs.

How do you determine what type and form of cannabis is right for your needs, as well as the potency and dose that's right for you? If your doctor or other health professional is knowledgeable about medical cannabis, it's wise to go over all of your options with that person. Another choice would be the advice of the budtender, who is the store's marijuana expert. If the budtender is experienced and well-informed, he should be able to steer you to several different options and assist you in choosing among them. I suggest allowing lots of time for your first few visits to the store so you can ask as many questions as necessary to be sure you get the best product that will suit your needs. And, of course, your own judicious research is also helpful; you can potentially get more targeted information in books and on the Internet on specific cannabis strains and products that may help with your health condition.

It will be fascinating to see the range of new strains and new cannabis products that will become available as laws become more progressive in various places around the globe. Entrepreneurs in the so-called "green rush" are eager to fill the needs of patients and, where it's legal, recreational users.

What About Growing Your Own Cannabis?

If you have a green thumb and the space and time for gardening indoors or outdoors, growing your own cannabis could be a wise and cost-effective decision—if you're legally allowed to do so in your jurisdiction. However, even if you are legally allowed to grow it, current laws may not allow you to grow enough for your needs. For example, if you're planning to juice raw cannabis, experts tell us it can take around 40 plants to supply the ongoing needs of one person. In the U.S., some of the states that allow medical marijuana do NOT allow patients to grow it. Others provide specific limits to the number of plants a patient may grow; a review of current state laws show ranges of 6 to 24 plants. State regulations can be accessed at http://medicalmarijuana.procon.org/view.resource.php?resourceID =000881.

The agricultural know-how required for your own garden of cannabis is beyond the scope of this book, but there's a lot of information available in books and online if this pursuit feels like an option for you.

What If Medical Cannabis Is STILL Not Legal Where You Live?

These days, many jurisdictions are no longer arresting people for possessing a small amount of cannabis. And, as I've shared, some companies are selling new high-CBD, very low-THC strains as nutritional supplements that are considered to be hemp, not medical marijuana. Because of this more relaxed atmosphere, some patients are more willing to risk buying cannabis on the street or growing their own. But if it's not legal in your part of the world, it may still be extremely risky.

I have heard recent stories of patients—and the parents of young patients—who have moved to another state or another country so they could legally obtain medical cannabis. I understand their motivation to do anything necessary to obtain medical cannabis because it's the one medication that has been the most helpful for me personally. Over the last few decades doctors and other health professionals have prescribed many medications and treatments for me, including both allopathic and alternative health options. While a couple of them have been very helpful, cannabis tops the list. I would do my best to move any- mountains that were in my way in order to obtain and use this healing herb.

Chapter 17

Understanding Potency and Quality Control

What does potency mean when we're talking about cannabis? Generally, we think of potency as the strength of a medicine. When you go to the store to purchase aspirin, you have a choice of two potencies—81 milligrams or 325 milligrams. You expect all of the brands of aspirin on the shelf to have the same chemical makeup, and you also expect each capsule or tablet to contain the exact amount of aspirin that's indicated on the label. In other words, aspirin is aspirin is aspirin—and the chemicals in it are basically the same no matter which brand you chose. But, because it's an herb, cannabis is different.

The chemical makeup of each cannabis strain is unique—containing a different amount of each of the 80 to 100 cannabinoids and the hundreds of other chemical compounds that are found in the plant. In fact, the ratio of these chemicals varies, not just from plant to plant, but also as the plant matures. If you harvest two leaves from the same plant at different times—even different times of the same day—it's probable that each leaf will have a slightly different chemical makeup.

Until medical cannabis is available with uniform labeling standards, it can be difficult to determine exactly what you're getting with any particular product. Each state or jurisdiction that has legalized medical marijuana has its own set of laws and rules about how it must be tested and labeled—and their requirements vary considerably, with few agreed-upon standards. As I discussed earlier in this book, most current labeling requirements are so minimal and insufficient that it's very difficult—and sometimes impossible—to compare cannabis products.

Everything possible should be done to make it clear to anyone who picks up a cannabis product that it is a cannabis product. That's true for any cannabis that you have in your home, including edibles such as candy and baked goods. To protect children, safety warnings should be noted on the label and childproof packaging should be standard. To date, my personal preferences have not included categories of cannabis edibles such as baked goods and candies. However, many people like taking cannabis that way, and that's great as long as they know the amount of cannabis that's in the edible product. Cannabis medicine is, after all, a *medicine*—and medicine should not be taken indiscriminately.

What should you consider in choosing cannabis products? When I first walked into a well-stocked medical marijuana collective, I was surprised to see the range of options in display cases, on shelves, and in the refrigerated and freezer sections. For those who want to smoke joints or use a pipe or bong, there were numerous jars of "buds," each containing a different strain. For those who prefer ways of ingesting cannabis other than smoking a joint or using a bong, the choices were also plentiful. They included vaporizers; various types of cannabis-filled capsules; tinctures; oral sprays in precision-dose atomizers similar to breath fresheners; and "edible" products that ranged from cannabis-infused cooking oils to cookies, candies, hot chocolate, coffee, and ice cream. There were also topical products—creams, salves, balms, and ointments.

Each person's unique body chemistry responds somewhat differently, so it can be challenging to pinpoint why one strain and type of cannabis is more healing for one than another. However, as you become a savvy medical marijuana patient, you will be better able to discern the information on a product's label and use that data in your selections. Be patient; it may take several tries to find a product that delivers the symptom relief that your body responds to or perhaps you will find a couple of products that, when taken together, work for you.

As I said before, each strain of cannabis has a unique chemical profile, composed of 80 to 100 cannabinoids AND hundreds of other chemicals. Many of these chemicals are present in such minute amounts that they fall below quantifiable levels. But they all count. Herbal medicine experts tell us that even those chemicals that show up in trace amounts have a role to play in the efficacy of that strain. After all, it is the synergy or entourage effect of all of the chemicals that's important.

You may experience little to no difference in symptom relief between two different cannabis products. Sometimes the difference is so subtle that it is not noticeable. On the other hand, in the same way I did, you may experience a major advantage from a new product overnight. At the beginning of this book, I mentioned experiencing huge improvement in a 25-year chronic cough after one day on a new high-CBD product. At that point in time, I had been taking a top quality cannabis product high in THC for a year and a half. It had helped me deal with other symptoms, but it did not quell that cough. Then, surprisingly, the day after I first took a high-CBD product, the cough become much less frequent. However, the high-CBD product didn't provide relief for my other symptoms, so I also continued taking the high-THC product.

Another issue with quality control is that the labs that test cannabis products often use different testing methodologies. It's not uncommon for growers and manufacturers to receive different results when samples from the same batch of product are tested at more than one lab—and I've learned that sometimes the results vary considerably. Many medical cannabis growers and manufacturers strive for the highest safety and quality standards—and they use respected labs that are aligned with those values. However, as with most industries, not every company in the medical cannabis world is motivated to follow high standards; some are focused on profit instead of quality. And the same is true with labs; I've heard of labs that "shop" high test results, skewing the numbers so they are the most advantageous to their customers.

Just as with any other medicine we consume, it's important that any given cannabis product contains what it purports to contain. In a study conducted by Steep Hill Halent of Colorado on behalf of *The Denver Post* and *The Cannabist*, edible cannabis products from a number of manufacturers were tested to determine how accurate their labels were. The shocking result was that only 25 percent of them—three products out of 12—were found to have the amount of THC that was listed on the label. In the case of one product, lab tests showed that it actually contained **less than one percent** of the amount of THC that was listed.[79]

At some point, it's probable—perhaps inevitable—that the U.S. will pass federal guidelines with across-the-boards standards for the growing, manufacturing, testing, and labeling of cannabis. Some medical cannabis pioneers are concerned that adding more government regulations will be too intrusive and make it even harder to do business—and I understand their concern. However, I also stand with other patients who depend on medical cannabis to relieve symptoms and potentially heal us, and feel it's critical that we actually get the quality and potency of medicine that we expect.

Chapter 18

Understanding the Different Types
of Cannabis Oil

Earlier in this book, I discussed the two types of cannabis products that are getting a lot of attention these days: cannabis oil and raw cannabis. In this chapter, we'll go into more depth on cannabis oil and, in the next chapter, we'll cover more on raw cannabis.

In this book, when I use the term *cannabis oil* I am referring to highly concentrated **medical cannabis** products, not the hemp oil that's available in your health food store next to the olive oil and canola oil. Cannabis oil is available in a syringe or small screw-top container. It can be taken on its own and is also available in products such as capsules, lozenges, ointments, and suppositories.

There are numerous products called cannabis oil, made from different strains of cannabis, each with very different ratios of cannabinoids, terpenes and flavonoids. Some are high in THC and can cause a great deal of psychoactivity. Others are low in THC but high in CBD. And still others, which are cold processed, contain THCa, a chemical in raw cannabis that has its own unique medicinal benefits and does *not* cause psychoactivity.

These cannabis oil products fit into two main types: *solvent extracted cannabis oil* and *cold processed cannabis oil*.

Solvent Extracted Cannabis Oil

When you are purchasing a cannabis oil product, it isn't always obvious what type of product it is. Until around 2013, most patients who used cannabis oil were using solvent-extracted oils that were high in THC. Then, the equivalent of a seismic shift occurred when cannabis oil made from new high-CBD strains became available. Some of these high-CBD strains also contain a considerable amount of THC, while other high-CBD strains contain only tiny amounts of THC and are therefore legally considered to be hemp, not cannabis, in most jurisdictions.

The process for making a solvent-extracted oil is complex and involves cooking the highly-flammable ingredients at a high temperature. Making this type of cannabis oil on your own is possible if you have the proper equipment. However, the directions for making this potent oil include danger warnings—since the slightest mistake can cause an explosion. These warnings are serious; I recently saw local television news reports of two different homes—in different parts of town—that blew up on the same night. Both explosions were blamed on illegal drug manufacturing in the homes. Maybe the individuals involved were new to the process—and maybe they were "cooking" something other than cannabis oil—however, even those who are sophisticated in these methods can make tragic mistakes.

Now let's look at the two categories of solvent-extracted cannabis oil—*high THC products that contain very little CBD* and *high CBD products that contain very little or no THC.*

A. Solvent-extracted high THC cannabis oil products, some of which contain very little CBD

Solvent-extracted cannabis oil used for medical purposes was popularized by a farmer in Canada, Rick Simpson. Simpson says that he cured his own skin cancer in 2003 after he learned how to make solvent-extracted cannabis oil, which he calls *hemp oil*. As I previously mentioned, in the U.S., the word *hemp* generally refers to non-psychoactive strains of cannabis that are used for industrial and food products. But, since cannabis is referred to as *hemp* in Canada, that's what Simpson calls it. At the time, almost all of the cannabis that was available was high in THC and very low in CBD. Therefore, most of the oils had little CBD content. After his own success, Simpson became a crusader, helping other patients by producing the oil and giving it away for free. Remarkably, he reports that since 2003 he has given this healing oil to over 5,000 patients who were dealing with many different types of cancer and other serious illnesses. Simpson's passion for helping people, fueled by the power of the Internet, morphed into a sort of ministry for him as he has shared this protocol in books and on websites and YouTube. Simpson, who has unfortunately spent time in prison for his medical cannabis work, has become a true international hero for the commitment he has made to share it with the world. It is clear from numerous reports posted on the Internet that Simpson has a special place in the hearts of many people who have been helped by his life-saving and brave generosity.

While I refer to the type of oil that Simpson makes as cannabis oil, it goes by a number of different names because, as manufacturers create their own versions of it, they call it by different product names. Many in the medical cannabis world pay homage to Simpson by referring to it as *Rick Simpson Oil*, *Simpson's Hemp Oil* or even the initials, *RSHO*, which stand for *Rick Simpson Hemp Oil*. However, not all that glitters is gold; I am aware of cannabis products that are of low or questionable quality that are called by confusingly similar names. As with most things in this world, it's up to you to use due diligence to assure that the cannabis products you buy are of the quality that you need and deserve.

Simpson says the feedback he has received from those who he supplied with cannabis oil indicates a success rate of 70 to 80 percent for those who followed his protocol. However, since it was totally illegal for him to share the oil with them and totally illegal for them to take it, Simpson also believes that many people who received his oil may have been afraid to contact him again—so the number of successes could be higher than 70 to 80 percent. Of course, it's unlikely that his true success rate will ever be known, but that doesn't matter to those who have been helped immeasurably because of his work.

In his book, *Nature's Answer for Cancer*, Simpson points out that healing can unfold quickly when a patient uses cannabis oil. For that reason, patients should carefully monitor their progress with their doctors since the dosage of other medications may need to be lowered or even eliminated. Simpson says:

> Patients should be aware of the fact that this oil can also reduce their blood pressure, ocular pressure, and blood sugar levels. If individuals are taking medications to treat these issues, they should be able to reduce their need for the use of the drugs they are currently using very rapidly in most cases. I must inform patients who take blood pressure medication that once they start the oil, often their blood pressure issues will no longer require the use of pharmaceuticals and this also holds true for diabetics and those who suffer with glaucoma as well.[80]

When treating cancer and other serious illnesses, many respected doctors and other experts use Simpson's protocol for cannabis oil (and products made from it) as their standard recommended treatment plan. This protocol is very specific and involves taking a very high dosage. In Chapter 21, I'll share the details of that protocol.

Simpson also advocates that healthy people take smaller amounts of the oil on a regular basis for its many benefits. In *Nature's Answer for Cancer*, he says:

> Everyone should be taking maintenance doses to keep their bodies detoxified and in a state of good health. All that is required is 1 to 2 grams of oil a month; just ingest a drop at night about an hour before bedtime. This will give you a good night's sleep .... The oil works with your body to keep you healthy and to provide protection from a wide variety of health issues.[81]

At the time that I switched to the more potent cannabis oil as my nighttime medicine, I had been taking capsules of cannabis extract every night for about five months. Two things happened almost immediately when I started taking the oil: First, I was more tired than ever; and second, I started losing weight at the rate of one-half to one pound a week without any changes to my diet or activity level. I didn't like the additional tiredness but, from a holistic perspective, I knew that it meant that the herb was probably causing my body to detox, which is ultimately a good thing. Think about any time when you were recouping from an injury or an illness; we almost always experience tiredness when we are in a healing mode.

In his videos and books, Rick Simpson explains that many patients who use this type of cannabis oil experience positive results regarding their weight—those who are overweight lose weight, while those who need to gain weight, gain weight. The amazing oil that has become synonymous with Simpson's name enabled him to easily lose 30 pounds. And many patients, including me, have had the same experience. I'm now closer to my ideal weight than I have been in a very long time.

B. High CBD products, some of which cause NO psychoactivity

High-CBD solvent-extracted cannabis oil products fall into two categories:

1. High-CBD cannabis oil that contains more than 0.3 percent THC, which may cause psychoactivity depending on the ratio of THC it contains and falls under marijuana laws in most jurisdictions

2. High-CBD cannabis oil and products made from strains that contain *almost no THC*, usually under 0.3 percent of the total cannabinoids, and do not cause psychoactivity

Solvent extracted high-CBD cannabis oil products are now becoming very popular with patients. As mentioned earlier, until recent years most cannabis oil products contained high amounts of THC, sometimes with little to no CBD. The newer cannabis oil products in this category contain much higher ratios of CBD than most patients had access to in the past. As an example of the second category above, an "almost no THC" strain might contain a ratio of 30 to 1 CBD to THC. Because there's so little THC in it, there's no psychoactivity associated with it, except in rare cases—and in many jurisdictions it is considered to be nutritional hemp, not marijuana. Therefore, laws pertaining to marijuana do not apply. However, as of this writing, this is still one of the gray areas regarding the legality of any cannabis product, so it's important that you check the regulations where you live.

An example of a high-CBD strain that contains less than 0.3 percent THC is Charlotte's Web™, which was developed by the Stanley Brothers of Colorado. Because CBD is known for its healing benefits, the Stanleys pioneered the breeding of new strains with a much higher ratio of CBD than that desired by recreational users. Their goal was to create a cannabis medicine that would be more efficacious for some patients. And they succeeded. The Stanleys were acclaimed for a high-CBD strain they bred that has been used to treat children with a condition called Dravet Syndrome, a specific type of epilepsy that causes debilitating seizures. As highlighted on the CNN documentary *Weed,* 5-year-old Charlotte Figi's seizures were reduced dramatically when she took the Stanleys' high-CBD product, which was named Charlotte's Web™ after her.

In addition to the Stanleys, other medical cannabis breeders and growers are now producing more new strains that are extremely high in CBD. Some of these strains are under 0.3 THC and, in many parts of the world, can be sold as nutritional supplements; while others are over 0.3 THC and are subject to medical marijuana laws.

Cannabis breeders and growers go through a complex process to develop strains that will be efficacious for patients; however, it's important to remember that the chemical profile of any specific strain may vary from crop to crop, depending on the stability of the strain itself and the specific growing conditions. After all, we're talking about a plant here, not a pharmaceutical product that is composed of chemicals that have been mixed together in specific proportions. It's also important to remember that not all patients will be helped by the same product, even when they have been diagnosed with the same condition.

I anticipate a day when patients will be able to access cannabis products that have a ratio of all of the plant's chemicals that are best for their unique needs—THC, CBD, the other cannabinoids, the terpenes, and the flavonoids. In the meantime, though, my own experience shows that experimenting with my protocol can improve the symptom relief that I experience. As new products have become available, trying them, tweaking the dosage, and sometimes combining them has provided even better results for me.

Cold Processed Cannabis Oil

Cold processed cannabis oil—the second category of cannabis oil products—is a newer trend that holds great promise for many because of its unique properties. Cold processed cannabis oil products are considered to be "raw" because the chemical THCa—a biosynthetic precursor to THC—is not heated and therefore, it is kept intact. As discussed earlier in this book and in the next chapter, THCa does not cause psychoactivity, except in very rare exceptions. Therefore, no matter what strain it is—or whether it is a high-CBD or high-THCa product—cold processed cannabis oil is not considered to be psychoactive.

Since cold processed cannabis oil also fits into the category of raw products, it is also discussed in the next chapter, "More on the Raw Cannabis Movement."

Chapter 19

More on the Raw Cannabis Movement

A form of cannabis that is leading to choruses of symptom relief from many—and remission from some—is raw cannabis. Raw cannabis can be juiced and is available from some manufacturers in capsules that contain raw cannabis oil or tablets made of the cold-processed whole plant. Another choice is to put raw cannabis leaves in a green salad; however, some patients find that it irritates the digestive tract.

From the perspective of a patient who doesn't want the high associated with cannabis, raw cannabis gives us another highly potent choice. But the biggest advantage of any raw cannabis product, from the perspective of someone who *doesn't want the high*, is this: Even if the strain of cannabis that's being used is high in THC, the psychoactive component, it will not lead to psychoactivity *as long as the cannabis has not been heated*. Whether it is being juiced or used in another form, the goal is to keep it from being exposed to *any* heat. Even an overheated motor on a juicer could potentially activate some of the THC and cause *some* degree of psychoactivity. And, because it can be difficult to avoid all sources of heat no matter how much care is taken, some raw cannabis products do contain a small amount of THC, although it is usually such a small amount that it is considered moot.

Dr. William Courtney is considered the pioneer of the raw cannabis juice movement. Dr. Courtney considers cannabis to be a superfood and calls it "... a dietary essential that helps all 210 cell types function more effectively." He says, "I don't even refer to it as medicine anymore, strictly as a dietary essential." Dr. Courtney's website, http://CannabisInternational.org, includes the following advice: "Cannabis provides highly digestible globular protein, which is balanced for all of the Essential Amino Acids. Cannabis provides the ideal ratio of omega 6 to omega 3 Essential Fatty Acids. Critically, cannabis is the only known source of the Essential Cannabinoid Acids. It is clear that all 7 billion individuals would benefit from access to cannabis as a unique functional food."[82]

The cannabinoid acids in raw cannabis products, including THCa and CBDa, work like NSAIDs (nonsteroidal anti-inflammatory drugs), reducing inflammation and modulating the immune system. However, as wonderful as raw cannabis products are for some patients, they do not provide symptom relief for everyone. Scientists believe that the *acid form* of cannabinoids, such as THCa and CBDa, are not efficacious for conditions that involve the CB1 and CB2 receptors, which are found mostly in the brain, spinal cord, immune system, and some other parts of the body. As more research is done, we'll know more about the conditions that are best treated with raw cannabis.[83]

Dr. Courtney's perspective on why fresh, raw cannabis should be considered as an important adjunct to any health regimen is also explained in this article by Leanne Dawson about his work:

> While Courtney understands that smoked cannabis can in fact be used as a medicinal therapy, he believes that in its best form, raw, it is a preventative. He claims cannabis is the "most important vegetable on the planet" and that it can assist the function of your immune system, provide anti-inflammatory benefits, and improve bone metabolism and neural function.

Cannabis is even capable of inhibiting cancer cell growth according to the doc; the list could go on and on.

According to the doctor, when you cook or smoke cannabis you are actually walking away from 99% of the benefits cannabis provides. Not to worry, in its raw form the plant contains THCa (Tetrahydrocannabinolic Acid) and CBDa (Cannabidiol Acid), which must be heated in order to produce THC and CBD.

Only when you decarboxylate THCa, turning it into THC, does it cause psychoactive effects or the "high" you may be used to when smoking cannabis. Additionally, the body is able to tolerate larger dosages of cannabinoids when cannabis is consumed in the raw form. This is because when you smoke cannabis, the THC actually acts as a CB1 receptor agonist and your body can only absorb about 10 mg at a time.

...Courtney suggests, "If you heat the plant, you will decarboxylate THC-acid and you will get 'high'. You'll get your 10mg (of THC). If you don't heat it, you can go up to five or six hundred milligrams, use it as a dietary cannabis and push it up to the anti-oxidant and neuro-protective levels which come into play at hundreds of milligrams. It is this dramatic increase in dose from 10 mg of psychoactive THC to the 500 mg—1,000 mg of non-psychoactive THCa, CBDA, and CBGA that comprises the primary difference between traditional 'Medical Marijuana' and Alternative Cannabinoid Dietary Cannabis."

The FDA has actually approved a tolerable CBD dose of 600 mg/day as a new investigative drug. This makes the medical potential of drinking the juice containing 600 mg of CBDA, far greater than when you heat the cannabis. Considering CBD percentages are typically below 1% in most strains, it would be physically impossible to smoke enough in one day to ingest a 600 mg dosage of CBD.[84]

To review, there are several reasons that raw cannabis products more efficacious for specific health conditions or symptoms:

1. Raw cannabis causes no psychoactivity, except in rare cases (which I'll address below)—and therefore works well for children as well as adults;
2. Raw cannabis contains the chemical THCa, which brings different and unique benefits to the table; and
3. Some raw cannabis products are also high in CBDa—the *acid* form of CBD, a biosynthetic precursor to CBD—which also has unique healing benefits.

Now let's look at raw cannabis in more detail. In its raw state, cannabis does not contain THC—except possibly in a very small, trace amount. Even strains of cannabis that are *high in THC when they are processed* contain little to no THC when they are raw. That's because the psychoactive-inducing chemical THC is not activated until cannabis is heated. Until cannabis is heated or dried, it doesn't contain THC; instead it contains THCa, which is a non-psychoactive chemical compound that is a biosynthetic precursor of THC. The "a" in THCa stands for the word "acid," so its full name is tetrahydrocannabinolic acid. When THCa is heated or dried, it is transformed into its psychoactive cousin, THC, through a chemical process called decarboxylation, which is also referred to as decarbing. In this process, water and carbon dioxide are released and the THCa becomes THC. *If THCa is not heated, it is still THCa. In almost ALL cases, this means it does NOT cause patients to experience psychoactivity.* However, there are two caveats:

1. A small amount of THC may be inadvertently converted
A very small "trace" amount of THCa may be converted into THC inadvertently in harvesting or processing, even when care is taken to avoid any heat; however, it is generally such a tiny amount that

it does not cause psychoactivity for most patients. The chemical profile of a raw cannabis oil capsule product that works well for me shows that its CBDa to THCa ratio is close to 3:1. However, it also contains very small amounts of CBD and THC, which means a small amount of the CBDa and THCa went through the process of decarboxylation, a chemical reaction that releases carbon dioxide (CO_2) and converts the CBDa to CBD and the THCa to THC. Here is the chemical breakdown as given on the label of that product; you may note that CBG, in both its acid and decarboxylated forms, is the only other cannabinoid listed:

> CBDa – 19.78 mg.
> CBD – 1.05 mg.
> THCa – 6.14 mg.
> THC – .87 mg.
> CBGa – 1.06 mg.
> CBG – .37 mg.

Since we know that most cannabis plants contain between 80 and 100 cannabinoids, it is likely that the ones found in this chemical profile—CBD, THC, and CBG, along with their "acid" form cousins, CBDa, THCa, and CBGa—are the only ones that are present in quantifiable amounts. Note that the decarboxylated forms of CBD and THC are both close to 1 mg.—with CBD at 1.05 mg. and THC at .87 mg. That's a very small amount. I am extremely THC sensitive; however, even my first time taking this product, I did not experience any psychoactivity.

I asked Rev. Dr. Kymron deCesare, the Chief Research Officer at Steep Hill Labs, for his opinion on the chemical composition of this particular capsule and he responded:

> There is NOT enough of any of the neutral cannabinoids in this capsule for those neutral cannabinoids to be

considered 'main ingredients,' ergo, they only work as entourage, or support function.

Effectively, this capsule contains approximately 27 mg. of cannabinoid acids, which are immune-modulating compounds. This capsule can be used to treat inflammation, pain resulting from inflammation, calming down the immune system when it overreacts (any kind of allergic reaction, poison oak, reaction to chemo-therapy, arthritis, etc.).

This specific capsule would be considered a 'moderate dose regimen.'[85]

2. In rare cases, THCa is converted to THC after it is ingested

Even when processed without heat, in some cases, the THCa in a cannabis product that is ingested could undergo "acid catalyzed decarboxylation" within the patient's stomach. Basically, that means the patient's own stomach acids catalyze the THCa and cause decarboxylation, thereby converting some THCa to THC. According to Rev. Dr. deCesare:

The degree of acid catalyzed decarboxylation a patient experiences depends on individual patient physiology. In most cases where it is reported, only a minor amount of THCa is decarboxylated, causing a mild psychoactive effect; while, in a very few patients, the effect is much larger. It is important that patients are warned of this infrequently occurring pharmacokinetic issue prior to treatment. The most often noticed psychoactive effect is a drop in cognitive processing (difficulty thinking, lack of focus). The Society of Cannabis Clinicians has done a good job of documenting this in case studies.[86]

If you are able to obtain an ongoing supply of fresh raw cannabis that is of high quality and free of mold and pesticide, I suggest you try juicing it. Just as with parsley and other herbs, cannabis doesn't yield a large amount of juice; therefore, it is best to use the type of juicer that is made for juicing wheat grass. Because of the bitter taste of cannabis, it needs to be mixed with other juices to make it palatable. One recommendation is to use at least ten parts vegetable and/or fruit juices to one part cannabis juice. There are a number of websites and YouTube videos that give instructions on raw cannabis juicing, including suggestions on the other juices to include in your recipe.

Raw cannabis should be ingested as soon as possible after it's been juiced because it oxidizes quickly, causing it to lose quality and turn brownish. Some experts suggest that the juice should be used within 12 hours in order to get the maximum benefit, while others say that it can be refrigerated for up to three days. Another option is to freeze the juice and use it right after unthawing it.

While raw cannabis juice may be the very best way to get the maximum benefit from cannabis, some experts point out that the cost is prohibitive for many patients. It's estimated that a patient needs 40 to 50 cannabis plants to have an ongoing supply for daily juicing. For that reason, the best option for those who are able to do so may be to obtain an appropriate strain of cannabis and grow your own.

When I started taking high-CBD raw cannabis oil capsules that were about a 3:1 CBDa to THCa ratio, I found two major benefits: 1) Since the capsules are made of raw cannabis oil, I do not experience any psychoactivity when taking them and can therefore take them at any time, day or night; and 2) Since I am able to take them in the daytime as well as during the night, I experience a reduction in both daytime and nighttime pain.

Chapter 20

What's the Best Cannabis Product for You?

If you are under the care of a health professional who works with cannabis patients, that person will be able to guide you on product choices and dosage. But it's still good to have an understanding of the options available to you. Also, since every individual's body responds somewhat differently to each new cannabis product, it's your responsibility to monitor the impact of any new medicine and report back to your health professional so they can best determine the most efficacious products and dose for your individual needs.

For those who do not have a medical cannabis expert to help with their decisions, understanding some basics about the selection of products and methods of administration is important. So let's look at what you need to consider in choosing the specific cannabis product or products that are right for you.

Cannabis Products with Little to No Psychoactivity

First of all, for those who want to avoid or limit the psychoactive effects of cannabis, let's review the types of cannabis products that produce little to no psychoactivity. Thankfully, for patients who do not want to experience the high or stoned feeling, many find effective options in three basic categories of cannabis products that contain only a very small amount of the psychoactivity-inducing chemical THC—or, possibly, none at all. While there are a couple of reasons, in rare circumstances, that *some* patients may experience *some* psychoactivity from these products, as I explain below, for the great majority of patients these products do not cause psychoactivity.

Cannabis medicine is in its infancy, so the jury is still out about the ratio of THC, other cannabinoids, terpenes, and flavonoids that will be best for various health conditions and symptoms. However, because CBD and the other cannabinoids work *with* THC, as well as all of the other chemical components of cannabis, it's unlikely that we should get rid of the THC—or any other compound in the plant—altogether. It's the ratio of all of the chemical compounds that we're concerned with because we want the most healing strain possible—and many patients also want the *most* efficacious product that causes the *least* amount of psychoactivity.

Here are the three broad categories of products that cause little to no psychoactivity:

- **High-CBD cannabis products that may be "legal everywhere"—well, almost everywhere, but subject to change**
  As regulations continue to catch up with what's already happening in both the medical and recreational marketplaces, what's legal today may be illegal tomorrow—and vice versa. In most jurisdictions, "legal everywhere" high-CBD cannabis is *very low* in THC—less than 0.3 percent. For those who respond better to low-THC products, a product in this category may be the best choice. Please note that many, if not most, of the cannabis strains that fit in this category also fit into the next category, nutritional products.

- **Nutritional products**

  Some cannabis supplements and other hemp products are categorized as nutritional rather than medical. As I discussed earlier, the word "hemp" can be confusing because it means different things to people in different parts of the world; however, many people use the word "hemp" to refer to the industrial strains of cannabis, which include food products and supplements. A few years ago, I started noticing hemp products, such as hemp milk and hemp seed oil, in the health food store. They have recently been joined by hemp protein products, as well as capsules, oils, extracts, and tinctures. These products are not categorized as marijuana because they contain only trace amounts of THC. But the amount of THC that's allowed is another gray area because, as of this writing, the U.S. government has not established standards for the amount of THC that is legally allowed in food products. However, because manufacturers are undoubtedly cautious about getting into legal wrangles with the government, it is likely that they contain less than 0.3 percent THC. Many products in this category are now available through online retailers, in health food stores, and over-the-counter in pharmacies.

- **Raw medical cannabis products**

  Raw cannabis does not produce psychoactivity, as it contains THCa and CBDa, the biosynthetic precursors to THC and CBD, which both have their own unique healing benefits. Raw cannabis can be made into fresh or frozen cannabis juice; eaten in a salad; and made into cold processed products including oil in a syringe, capsules, or tablets.

Routes of Administration and Product Choices

The way the cannabis is delivered or ingested, which is referred to as the "route of administration," determines the speed and efficiency with which it is absorbed by the body, how long it takes until symptom relief sets in, and how long those effects last. We want the maximum medicinal benefit from any cannabis product we take, and the route of administration can greatly impact the benefit we derive from it. That's why I created the next chart, which presents your cannabis options according to the ways each type of product is administered, the length of time it takes for the onset of its effect, and the potential duration period.

I have divided the route of administration into five categories— inhalation or vaping, gut absorption, oral mucosal delivery, suppositories, and topical products. Obviously, some types of cannabis products, like a vape-pen or a cannabis cookie, can only be administered in one specific way since your only choice is to inhale through the vape-pen and eat the cookie. The same is true for suppositories and topical products, which only have one possible delivery method. However, some savvy medical marijuana patients find that they can achieve faster symptom relief by taking products in an alternative way. For instance, instead of swallowing a capsule, which may take an hour or two for the onset of symptom relief, capsules can bring symptom relief in seconds or minutes if they are placed in the mouth and allowed to melt into the mucosal lining of the mouth, which is often referred to as the oral mucosa.

Routes of Administration and Product Choices			
Delivery Method	**Product Choices** Note that some products can be delivered via more than one delivery method	**Onset Time**	**Duration of Effect**
Inhalation or Vaping	•Joints •Pipes and bongs •Vape-pens	Almost immediate	Varies considerably; up to 3 hours
Gut absorption	Any product that is *swallowed or chewed*, including: •Capsules or tablets •Cannabis oil in syringes or small screw-top containers •Extracts, tinctures, and oral sprays •Raw cannabis leaves, juiced or in a salad •Soft, chewable candies such as chocolates, lozenges, and gummy-bears; baked goods; ice cream; and other cannabis-infused foods •Cannabis drinks, including specialty drinks, teas, hot chocolate, and coffee	1 to 2 hours	Up to 8 hours
Oral Mucosal	•Capsules •Cannabis oil in syringes or small containers •Extracts, tinctures, sprays •Soft, chewable candies and foods such as chocolates, lozenges, and gummy-bears	From seconds to 15 minutes	Up to 8 hours
Suppositories	•Cannabis suppositories—already made or made at home with a kit •Cannabis capsules used as suppositories	Varies	Varies
Topical Products	•Cannabis-infused creams, salves, balms, ointments, transdermal patches •Cannabis oil in syringes or small screw-top containers	Varies	Varies

Now let's look at each of these methods of administration in greater detail:

Inhalation or Vaping

Product Choices: Joints, pipes, bongs, vape-pens
Onset Time: Almost immediate
Duration of Effect: Varies; up to 3 hours

Smoking a joint or using a pipe or bong are the age-old ways of inhaling cannabis and these are the methods that most people associate with the herb. The inhalation route of administration is great for fast symptom relief and a wide variety of strains is available in most marijuana stores. While some of the cannabis smoke or vapor is immediately absorbed by the mucosal membranes in the mouth, most of it goes directly into the bloodstream via the lungs. Most patients notice the effects within three to ten minutes—and that fast relief can be important for people who are suffering from nausea, the rapid onset of a migraine headache, anxiety, or a host of other issues. Fast onset is a big advantage to any inhalation method; however, there is a trade-off because the beneficial effects are of much shorter duration than other methods.

Today's patients who prefer to inhale their cannabis medicine also have a newer option—vaporizers that utilize the same technology as e-cigarettes. Because of their size and shape, these electronic devices are often referred to as *vape-pens* or *pen vaporizers*. There's no smoke involved since vaporizers produce an odorless vapor. They are powered by a lithium ion rechargeable battery and come with a charging device that fits into a USB port on a computer or in a wall socket. The vape-pen holds a small cartridge that's filled with cannabis oil. When the user puffs on the vape-pen, a small drop of the oil is released from the cartridge and heated, causing it to volatilize or evaporate into a pure odorless vapor, which is then inhaled as a fine mist. Vape-pens were considered by some to be the "cleanest" method of inhalation; however, recent concerns have been raised about the ingredients that are mixed with the cannabis oil in vape-pen cartridges. Also, as with all cannabis products, it's important that the cannabis oil inside the cartridge be a strain that is efficacious for you, of high quality, preferably organic, and without any toxic residue or questionable additives.

In his online article, "How Safe Is Your Vape Pen?," Jahan Marcu, PhD points out that "... there may be a hidden downside to vape pens, which are manufactured (typically in China), marketed, and utilized without regulatory controls. Available online and in medical marijuana dispensaries, vape pens contain a battery-operated heating mechanism, which at high temperatures can transform solvents, flavoring agents, and various vape oil additives into carcinogens and other dangerous toxins."[87]

Marcu specifically addresses his concern about one common additive to many vape-pen cartridges, a chemical called propylene glycol, a humectant (used to keep moisture in products), solvent, and preservative in food and tobacco products. Even though the U.S. Food and Drug Administration classifies it as "generally recognized as safe" for ingestion and topical use, many holistic health experts are wary of its safety in general. And many are even more concerned when it's added to cannabis oil that's going to be vaporized because of the question of how the heat might affect this chemical and possibly make it dangerous to breathe. Also, a recent news story reported that a vape-pen blew up in a man's hand, causing the loss of the tip of a finger, as well as damage to his face. Is this kind of accident due to the lack of manufacturing standards—or should we be concerned about a device that combines a battery and heat and, perhaps, potentially toxic ingredients that can be off-gassed? The jury is out so I suggest that you do further research before deciding to buy one.

When I first became a medical cannabis patient, the idea of inhaling it—through any means—wasn't a match for me. I preferred to use edible products such as capsules and lozenges because I liked the idea of getting a precise dose every time I took cannabis. But I eventually found that a vape-pen came in handy at times. **At the moment, I no longer use a vape-pen because of the aforementioned concerns about toxicity from the ingredients that are mixed with the cannabis and the heat from the device itself which might make potentially toxic ingredients even more toxic.** However, I like the idea of keeping the door open for this method of inhalation in the event a way is found to assure patients that it i-s safe.

Whether smoking, using a bong or pipe, or a vape-pen, these inhalation methods can be helpful due to the quick onset they provide. When I did use a vape-pen, I found it helpful in the timing of my nighttime regimen. I take my overnight dose of cannabis oil, lozenge, or tincture spray about an hour before bed. However, on evenings that I get home late, I have a timing issue because it takes an hour to two hours until the cannabis relaxes my body so I can sleep. In the past, on nights like that I would take the cannabis as soon as I got home and then stay up until I started to feel some effect from the medicine or go to bed and lay there for quite a while, until I finally drifted off into sleep. Either way, sleep was deferred while my body absorbed the cannabis. I have to admit that the vape-pen came in handy on such occasions because, while the edible product was being absorbed, I would get settled in bed and take some puffs. With any inhalation method, taking the puffs slowly and holding the vapor in the mouth as long as possible allows the mucous membrane lining inside the mouth—called the oral mucosa—to absorb as much of it as possible before the rest of it travels to the lungs to be absorbed there.

If you are new to inhaling, it can take some getting used to. When I first started using a vaporizer, I had to get used to puffing it. Vaping wasn't as easy as I thought it would be—probably because I didn't know how to inhale. Honest! But, with a minimal amount of practice, I'm now pretty good at it.

Gut Absorption

Product Choices: Any product that is *swallowed or chewed*, including:
- Capsules or tablets
- Cannabis oil in syringes or small screw-top containers
- Extracts, tinctures, and oral sprays
- Raw cannabis leaves, either juiced or in a salad
- Soft, chewable candies such as chocolates, lozenges, and gummy-bears; baked goods; ice cream; and other foods
- Cannabis drinks, including specialty drinks, teas, hot chocolate, and coffee

Onset Time: 1 to 2 hours
Duration of Effect: Up to 8 hours

Some medical cannabis experts refer to any product that is absorbed through the gut as an *edible*, whether it's a cannabis-infused brownie that you eat or a capsule that you swallow. Other experts divide foods and capsules into different categories; however, since both categories involve gut absorption, I'm discussing both in this section.

One of the main benefits of any product that travels through your digestive system *before* entering your bloodstream is the longer duration of symptom relief, which can last up to eight hours. The drawback to gut absorption is the onset time since it usually takes an hour or two before a patient feels the herb's effect. That's why it's so important to start with a very small amount of any new product.

Before it can go to work, cannabis that you take through the gut has to be absorbed through the body's long and winding gastrointestinal tract, go through the liver, and then be metabolized. It takes an hour or two to be absorbed, before allowing the patient to finally feel its effects. The same is true for any medication that you take orally; it always takes a while until it impacts the body. But the wait is worth it because the beneficial effects often last six hours or longer, making it a preferred way to take cannabis for those who desire a longer period of symptom relief.

Since it takes longer to feel the effects of cannabis products that are absorbed through the gut, it's important to start with a small dose and allow up to two hours to determine how it affects you before taking more. A person who doesn't feel the impact of the medicine— and then takes more too soon—might easily over-medicate. This caution is especially important if the cannabis product you're taking is one that contains more than a tiny amount of THC and, therefore, causes at least some degree of psychoactivity, except perhaps for those who have built up a tolerance to it over time.

Over-medicating on cannabis that's taken through the gut can happen before you know it. In a *New York Times* op-ed, journalist Maureen Dowd relates an experience she had while reporting on the legalization of recreational marijuana in Colorado. She ate a small piece of a pot-laced candy bar, felt no reaction to it, and then ate more. After about an hour, Dowd *really* felt the effects. She experienced hallucinations and paranoia that lasted for an eight-hour period, during which she was unable to move from the bed. Dowd later learned that, for novices, the cannabis candy bar was supposed to be cut into 16 pieces, each of which represented one "dose." However, she said there were no instructions about the size of a dose on the label.[88] Unfortunately, overdosing happens all too frequently, especially in places where few labeling requirements exist.

Thankfully, producers of edible cannabis products are now starting to add more dosage information on labels, especially in jurisdictions where new regulations now require them to do so. However, since the word "dose" in this context is very unclear—and may vary from manufacturer to manufacturer—I would advise a newcomer to cannabis to be extremely cautious. Unless you know for sure that the "dose" is within your own tolerance limits, I suggest starting with a *really* tiny amount—perhaps one-tenth of a dose. If you don't feel any effects within two hours, you can always take more. But if you take too much, you'll have to ride the full wave of the psychoactivity, which might take a day or more and could include a negative "trip." Eventually, you'll find a dose that seems to maximize symptom relief and other benefits and you can stay there until you want to increase or decrease it.

While ingesting cannabis through the gut provides longer-lasting benefits, it's generally not as efficient as other methods for three reasons:

1. Onset takes longer than inhaling, vaping, or using products that are taken via the oral mucosa
2. The absorption rate may vary depending on the amount of undigested food in the stomach when it is taken
3. Some people simply have more efficient digestive systems that are better at absorption than others

Let's look at the categories of cannabis products that are swallowed and absorbed through the gut in more detail. Also, note that some of these products can, alternatively, be taken via other routes of administration.

Capsules: Gelatin capsules come in two types—hard-shelled capsules with two halves that are each filled with medication and then joined together and soft capsules made from one continuous piece of gelatin that encapsulates the medication. While hard-shelled capsules are more common in the medical cannabis world, some soft gel capsule products are available. Traditionally, gelatin capsules are not vegetarian; however, some manufacturers use vegetarian gelatin capsules. Because the THC in cannabis is only soluble in a fat, some type of fat is included in the capsules to activate it, such as grapeseed oil, coconut oil, or butter. There are two basic types of cannabis capsules:

- **Cannabis Oil Capsules:** These capsules contain cannabis oil that is produced through solvent extraction or cold processing as described earlier in this chapter.
- **Cannabis Extract Capsules:** A second type of capsules are made from a whole plant extract that is heat processed without using a solvent, such as one company's product, Cannabis Extract Whole Plant Capsules. Because the content of these capsules is dense, not runny like the oil in cannabis oil capsules, it's possible to cut them apart and take a small portion if you want a smaller dose.

Tablets: To date, I am aware of only one type of cannabis tablet—a cold processed whole plant tablet. Because it is cold processed, this tablet is in the category of raw cannabis.

Cannabis oil in syringes or small screw-top containers: The oil, which is fairly thick, can be squeezed into the mouth and swallowed or put onto a tortilla chip, cracker, tiny piece of bread, or other "carrier," and then eaten. However, as with other products, its onset is much faster when administered via the oral mucosa and allowed to dissolve there instead of via the gut. (Also see "Oral Mucosal Delivery" below.) Some patients find it challenging to take cannabis oil in this form due to its bitterness, which can be difficult for the stomach and cause queasiness, especially when you increase to a high dose. That's why some companies are manufacturing other types of products that contain cannabis oil, such as gummy bears or lozenges, which are more palatable.

As you'll learn in more detail in the next chapter on protocols, patients who are new to cannabis should start with a teeny, *tiny* dose. This caution is even more important when you are taking cannabis oil because it can be challenging to get *an exact dose* from a syringe or container—and therefore, it can be easy to overdose. When I suggest taking a "teeny, tiny" dose, I mean it. Think of the size of *half* of a piece of short-grain, uncooked rice, and start there. Then, over time, increase the amount. If your protocol involves taking a much larger dose on a regular basis, most experts suggest doubling the dose every three or four days until you get to the desired dose.

Most syringes are available in one gram (1,000 milligrams) and five gram (5,000 milligrams) sizes and they have marks on the side that indicate the dosage, allowing the patient to squeeze out the desired amount. There are ten doses of 100 milligrams in a one gram syringe—and there are ten indicator marks on the side that tell you exactly how much oil equals a 100 milligram dose; therefore, it's generally pretty easy to squeeze out the amount you want with a fair degree of precision. But if you have a five gram syringe and you want a 100 milligram dose, you need to squeeze out one-fiftieth of the contents—and doing that with accuracy is trickier.

Another factor in using cannabis oil that comes in a syringe or screw-top container is its viscosity or ease of flow, which is impacted by temperature and, in some areas, humidity. Like most cannabis products, this oil should be refrigerated. However, when the oil is cold, it's even more difficult to dose a precise amount. You may find that taking the syringe out of the refrigerator five minutes before you plan to use it will make it easier to squeeze out the amount you desire.

If necessary, when squeezing the oil from a syringe, use a toothpick to guide the ribbon of oil and maneuver it onto an implement or a bite of food as a "carrier." I have used a number of different carriers for cannabis oil, including the back of a spoon, a popsicle stick, a bite-sized corner of a slice of bread, a cracker, and a tortilla chip. Of these choices, my preference is the tortilla chip. I squeeze the oil onto a small corner of a chip, then bite the oil-laden corner off the chip and hold it in the back of my mouth, between my jaw and my cheek. Within a minute or two, the small piece of tortilla chip dissolves in my mouth. By allowing it to dissolve this way, I am combining gut absorption with oral mucosal delivery, as described below, for faster absorption. If you decide to try using bread as a carrier, you may find, as I did, that the cold oil caused the piece of bread to crumble as I attempted to maneuver the oil onto it. My solution was to use a very small corner of a slice of frozen bread because its harder surface made it easier to convey the oil onto it.

No matter how you ingest cannabis oil, because of its messy, sticky nature, any oil residue on your teeth, tongue, or gums can't easily be rinsed away. And even if you could rinse it away, you wouldn't want to do so because you get the most benefit from it when you allow the oil to be slowly absorbed into your system through the oral mucosa. Should any of the gooey stuff get on your fingers, I suggest you do what I do and lick it off, taking as much time as necessary to do a thorough job of it because, despite the fact that it tastes bitter, this stuff is like gold in terms of its value. However, if you want to quickly remove it, rubbing alcohol can be used, but a soapy washcloth or paper towel also does the trick if you have a bit of patience and tenacity about it.

Extracts, tinctures, and oral sprays: An extract, tincture, or oral spray product that is immediately swallowed will be absorbed mostly through the gut. The alternative is to hold the liquid in the mouth as long as possible so more of it will be absorbed by the oral mucosal lining, providing faster onset.

Raw cannabis leaves, either juiced or in a salad: Gut absorption is the only way to ingest cannabis juice or leaves that have been added to a salad.

Soft, chewable candies such as chocolates, lozenges, and gummy-bears; baked goods; ice cream; and other foods: Any cannabis based candy or food that can be chewed and swallowed can be administered via gut absorption. However, for quicker onset of benefits, some types of candies can also be taken via oral mucosal delivery; see "Oral Mucosal Delivery of Edible Products" below. With the exception of some very hard candies, the advantage of most of the products in this category is that they can easily be cut into smaller doses with a knife or kitchen scissors. For example, I prefer "soft lozenges," which are similar to gummy bear-type candy, to oil in a syringe because it's much easier to take exactly the dose I desire—and the gummy bear taste disguises the bitterness of the oil to some extent. Lozenges that contain 250 milligrams of cannabis can easily be cut with a knife or kitchen scissors. If you want to take 125 milligrams, it's easy to cut the lozenge in half. Then, if you want an even smaller dose, you can continue cutting it into smaller pieces. For example, if you want a dose of 25 milligrams, cut each half of the lozenge into five pieces that are approximately the same size. They won't each be precisely 25 milligrams, but will probably be fairly close. Please note: Some products may be easier to cut if the knife or scissors is hot; simply heat the implement by putting it in a cup of hot water or holding it under running hot water for a minute or so.

Cannabis drinks, including specialty drinks, teas, hot chocolate, and coffee: A wide variety of cannabis drinks are available. If you savor each gulp in your mouth before swallowing it, a small amount of the cannabis will be absorbed via your oral mucosa; however, the majority will be absorbed in the gut.

Oral Mucosal Delivery

Product Choices: Any cannabis product that is ingested through the lining of the mouth or under the tongue, including capsules

Onset Time: From seconds to 15 minutes

Duration of Effect: Up to 8 hours

Whether it is a tincture, extract or spray, or even a gummy-bear type candy that you allow to melt in your mouth, you get more benefit from the product when it is delivered to the mucosal membranes that line the inside of the mouth *or* sublingually, under the tongue, on the floor of the mouth. When you hold the cannabis product inside your cheeks or under your tongue for as long as possible before swallowing, delivery to the bloodstream is much faster and the beneficial effects last much longer than through inhalation. Oral mucosal delivery can be used for any cannabis product that can be held in the mouth or under the tongue long enough so that some or all of it is absorbed by the mucosal membranes.

The longer you're able to hold the cannabis product in your mouth, the more you will absorb through the oral mucosa. While it is probably certain that *some* of the product will escape down your throat and be absorbed through your digestive system, the more of any edible product that is absorbed through the oral mucosa, the faster you will experience the desired benefits. The only drawback in taking cannabis medicine in this manner is the taste of these products, which can be very bitter in some cases.

Products that can be taken through the oral mucosa include:

Cannabis Oil Capsules: While we generally think of swallowing capsules, they can be ingested via the oral mucosa instead. Simply place a capsule inside the mouth, between the gums and the inside of the cheek, and hold it there until the gelatin covering melts. The oil will then be released in your mouth. An alternative method is to place the capsule in the back of the mouth between two teeth and then carefully bite down just enough to pierce the capsule in one place with a tooth, allowing the oil inside to slowly ooze out. Whichever method you use, do your best to hold the oil in your mouth as long as possible rather than swallowing it. I feel that this second method gives me an even faster onset of benefits, probably because more of the oil is absorbed in the oral mucosa and less of it inadvertently goes down the throat. But be forewarned—most cannabis oils are quite bitter, so if you try this method, be prepared for that. As far as I'm concerned, it's worth it.

Cannabis Extract Capsules: Hard-shelled gelatin capsules that contain whole extract cannabis mixed with a fat such as organic butter can be also taken via the oral mucosa instead of being swallowed. The capsule is placed inside the mouth, between the gums and the inside of the cheek, and allowed to melt there. It may take a while, but the gelatin will dissolve and the contents will disperse in your oral cavity. Because the cannabis mixture in the capsule is so dense, this type of capsule can be frozen, which makes it easy to cut into smaller, fairly uniform-sized pieces on a cutting board, allowing for more precise dosing if you don't want to take the entire capsule. I keep one Sativa capsule and one Indica capsule in the freezer at all times. Then, whenever I want, I have the option of a smaller dose because I can easily remove the gelatin "skin" of the capsule and place a small blob of the cannabis mixture directly onto the oral mucosa, where it dissolves fairly quickly. However, I don't keep more than one or two of each type of capsule in the freezer because once they've been frozen, they must remain frozen until they are ingested. I learned that lesson the hard way when I left a frozen capsule on the kitchen counter and later found that it had defrosted into a gooey gelatinous mess, which was impossible to swallow. It's certainly fine to keep your gelatin capsules in the freezer if you want; just remember that frozen capsules (or pieces of them) need to be used right out of the freezer; you can't thaw them out and put them in a container for future use unless you want a mess on your hands.

Cannabis oil in a syringe or small screw-top container: The onset time for cannabis oil is much faster when administered via the oral mucosa and allowed to dissolve there instead of traveling through the gut. When the oil is slowly delivered to the body in this way, via the oral mucosa, more of it enters the bloodstream, making it a more effective delivery system. However, the downside of taking cannabis oil in this way is that it can be extremely bitter, which is especially challenging for those who need to ingest a large dose. There are several ways of ingesting cannabis oil through the oral mucosa. Some patients simply do whatever is necessary to apply the sticky stuff to the inside of one of the cheeks and hold it there as long as possible. Another method is to put the oil on a hard piece of candy and then stick the candy in your mouth and slowly suck on it until it is dissolved. Or you can deposit the oil sublingually, which simply means placing it under the tongue to be absorbed by the body. On the website http://420magazine.com another method to deliver cannabis oil to the oral mucosa is nicely described. Referred to as the "tacking" method, it involves applying a drop of the oil onto your index finger and then applying it in various spots on the bottom area of your gums.[89] Whichever method you use, you will achieve faster onset and maximize its benefits the more slowly it is absorbed.

Extracts, tinctures, and oral sprays: An extract, tincture, or oral spray product that is immediately swallowed will be absorbed mostly through the gut. The alternative is to hold the liquid in the mouth as long as possible so more of it will be absorbed by the oral mucosal lining, providing faster results.

Soft, chewable candies and foods such as chocolates, lozenges, and gummy-bears: Any edible that you are able to hold in your mouth for more than a second or two may benefit you more quickly if at least a portion of it is dissolved in your mouth, rather than through the digestive tract. There are no rules for oral mucosal delivery; however, a chewy brownie may or may not dissolve there, so use your judgment. Simply try it out if it feels possible with any specific product. Instead of chewing the product, hold it in the side of the mouth, between the teeth and the inside of the cheek, as long as possible to allow it to "melt" and dissolve.

Suppositories

Product Choices: Cannabis suppositories can be purchased or made at home using a kit; also, cannabis capsules used as suppositories

Note: As of this writing, limited research is available about the onset time or duration of effect of cannabis medicine that is administered as a suppository. Both the potency and dosage of the cannabis will, of course, be factors.

Suppositories, which are inserted into the rectum, are a viable option for patients who have conditions related to the colon or those for whom other methods of administration are not possible due to nausea or other complications. The mucosal lining of the colon and the rest of the digestive system is thin, allowing for quick absorption into the bloodstream.

Cannabis suppositories are available in some marijuana stores or you can purchase a suppository kit and make your own cannabis suppositories. Another option that some people find effective is to insert a gelatin cannabis capsule like a suppository; however, I understand that not all gelatin capsules dissolve well so some trial and error may be required.

Suppository kits can be purchased at health food stores, homeopathic pharmacies, and through online merchants. The kits include instructions, molds, and a "carrier," such as beeswax, which is mixed with cannabis and then inserted into the molds. You can use raw cannabis that's been ground into a fine powder, cannabis oil, or cannabis extract. A friend learned that cannabis can be delivered to the body through suppositories and decided to add that protocol to her regimen. She bought a suppository kit, added some cannabis oil to the equation, and found that making her own was easy. When she used a suppository before bed, she said she knew it was doing its good work during the night because even a tiny burp in the morning had a cannabis after-taste to it. Clearly, the herb was working its way through her body and doing its thing.

Topical Products

Product Choices: Cannabis-infused creams, salves, balms, ointments and transdermal patches; cannabis oil in syringes or small screw-top containers

Note: Topical products are applied directly to specific areas of the body; onset time and duration of effect will vary from product to product.

There are numerous medical cannabis products available in the form of creams, salves, balms, ointments and transdermal patches that are designed to be used directly on the skin. Additionally, cannabis oil from a syringe or small screw-top container and products made from it can also be applied as a topical medication and have been touted by Rick Simpson for healing his own skin cancer, as discussed in the previous chapter. Topical cannabis products are generally used directly on the areas of the body that are impacted by pain, inflammation, or muscle spasms, while others are touted as the newest trend in anti-aging beauty and skin products. If you are treating a specific area of the body, if possible, apply a layer of the product and then cover the area with a bandage to allow the medicine to be absorbed over time. Another method of administration for a topical cannabis product is to massage it onto the soles of the feet. According to the principles of Chinese foot reflexology, this method transports the medicine to the entire body through the acupuncture points—allowing for additional benefits.

Chapter 21

How to Determine the Best Protocol for You

After reading this book, I hope that any stigma or concern you might have about medical cannabis will have evaporated. As it becomes more accepted and appreciated around the world, I also hope that more people will have easy and affordable access to it and that each patient will have specific and clear guidelines on the best protocol for their needs. But, until that happens, most patients will have to determine their own protocol.

It is very important that the cannabis you obtain is of a high quality. In addition to the standards that are essential to proper growing and harvesting, cannabis products that go through a manufacturing process must also be prepared properly. To that end, because cannabis is not water-soluble, some forms or types of products require either an alcohol base or a fat base—using "good" fats such as organic butter, olive oil, and coconut oil—so the body can best utilize the medicine.

When cannabis is smoked or vaporized, the onset of effects is fairly rapid—usually within three to ten minutes. That rapid onset is important to some patients—but the downside with smoking joints or using a vaporizer is the much shorter duration of the symptom relief. Nevertheless, puffing on a joint or vape-pen one or more times daily may be all that is needed for some patients who are in pain, experiencing anxiety, or dealing with any number of other symptoms or conditions. Those who are looking for longer-lasting relief may decide to use cannabis in capsules, tablets, and other edibles. Even though it usually takes an hour or two to feel the beneficial effects from an edible product, those effects can last for as long as six to eight hours, depending on the quantity that's been taken and the tolerance the patient has developed. And some patients find that a combination of products provides the most benefits.

Tolerance—and Titrating Your Dosage

In the context of medicines, *tolerance* means that the body starts to "tolerate" or become used to the effects of a medicine as we continue to take it. In essence, the medication works for a while to ease or quell symptoms and then, as the body adapts to the medication and starts to depend on it, the dosage and/or potency needs to be increased to get the same desirable effects. But, in the medical cannabis world, the word tolerance is often used in a slightly different context since most people think of it in relationship to a patient's ability to deal with the psychoactive high or stoned feeling of THC. As we covered in Chapter 14, "What About Potential Side Effects and Psychoactivity?", over time, as their bodies develop a tolerance to cannabis, many—if not most—patients find that they no longer experience effects that they find undesirable.

Patients need to monitor their tolerance to cannabis, as well as the extent to which they are benefiting from each cannabis product they're taking. At this point in time, most patients don't have access to the guidance of a doctor or other health professional who is an expert in cannabis medicine, so they also have to *self-titrate*. That means they must determine what specific cannabis product to take, in what quantity and at what intervals, as well as when to increase (or decrease) their dosage in order to continue to get the same degree of symptom relief—or more symptom relief. This is very different from what we're used to with pharmaceutical drugs. When your doctor gives you a prescription, she monitors the impact of that drug on you over time. If she feels you are benefiting from the medication and wants you to continue taking it, she may *titrate*—or adjust—your dosage upward or downward.

Until recently, it was difficult for patients to avoid the psycho-active effects of cannabis because most of the products that were available contained a high ratio of THC. However more and more low-THC products, which cause little to no psychoactivity, have come on the market—and, of course, that includes raw cannabis products, which cause NO psychoactivity at all. However, I must add a caveat here because some conditions may require a high-THC strain.

If a cannabis product that does not cause psychoactivity is efficacious for you, you can focus on symptom relief and healing without having to factor in the psychoactive effects. However, since each patient builds tolerance to the various effects of cannabis at different speeds, you still need to titrate your dosage carefully in order to get the maximum healing potential. Those who are new to cannabis should start with a very small dose and then slowly increase it over a period of time as their level of tolerance builds. However, if a patient has been a frequent user of marijuana in the past, he may already have a higher level of tolerance than most people and, therefore, it may be appropriate for him to start at a higher dose in order to get the efficacy he wants and needs.

When a high degree of tolerance is achieved, patients who are taking psychoactive forms of cannabis often find the side effects of the "high," such as psychoactivity, are greatly diminished. However, the patient still benefits from the all of the medicinal effects, such as control of pain, nausea, insomnia, muscle spasms, etc. At that point, the positive effects continue and the patient can continue taking cannabis without needing to increase the dosage. For some patients, that level may come in days or weeks, while for others it may take months of tweaking the type of product and dosage to get the maximum benefits.

If you feel groggy in the morning after taking cannabis the night before, you may be taking too much and want to consider lowering your dosage—at least until your tolerance increases. However, with some protocols, grogginess may be unavoidable. If you have a serious health challenge and decide to follow the high-dosage protocol developed by Rick Simpson, which is detailed later in this chapter, you will be taking 60 grams of cannabis oil over a period of 90 days, starting with a very small dose and then doubling it every three to four days, until you are taking one gram a day. If you are following a high-dose protocol like Simpson's, you may feel groggy lot of the time and you must adjust your lifestyle accordingly. If possible, check with your doctor or medical cannabis advisor to determine your own best protocol.

Because each person responds to cannabis in different ways, we have to use common sense, trial and error, and any other viable methods to determine how much cannabis medicine any individual should take. Unless patients are given a specific protocol by a doctor or other health practitioner, there are a host of questions that we have to find our own answers for:

- Which form of cannabis product is the best for me—smoking, vaporizing, edibles, suppositories, creams or salves?
- Should I use more than one product concurrently?
- If the cannabis product I select is available in both indica and sativa, which should I choose?
- Is there a "right" amount that will give me the maximum benefit?

The doctor who signed your medical marijuana paperwork has simply given you legal access to cannabis in the forms and types that your local jurisdiction allows. Perhaps it's different in some places – and, of course, medical marijuana laws are in a state of flux—but, as I'm writing this, doctors who prescribe cannabis in some states and jurisdictions are not legally allowed to tell their patients which strains to use, which forms or types to use, or what potency they should take. For many patients, the clerk in a medical cannabis shop—called a budtender—is the only person available to answer these questions and give specific recommendations.

Some budtenders are very knowledgeable about medical cannabis, know their product inventory well, and do a good job of recommending the best options for each patient. Depending on your situation, a knowledgeable budtender may be able to help you select the best cannabis products for your needs. But if you have a serious health issue—either acute or chronic—the budtender may not be the best advisor for you and it's also possible that his shop might not carry the forms or types of cannabis that are best to treat your condition.

Budtenders are similar to pharmacists in some ways. But, among the many distinctions between them, pharmacists simply fill a prescription *exactly* the way your doctor prescribed it. If you request counseling, a pharmacist will counsel you on the drug involved. But the prescription is for a very specific drug at a very specific potency and with a very specific dosage that your doctor prescribed; the pharmacist cannot suggest a medication that your doctor didn't prescribe or even a different dosing schedule. On the other hand, the budtender can help the medical marijuana patient select from a whole store full of different cannabis products, including many different strains of cannabis buds for smoking or vaporizing. The patient is then "allowed" to purchase any one of them, sometimes with a limit on the quantity that can be purchased.

While some budtenders are quite knowledgeable, how do you know if they are giving you the best information for your own health needs? I have visited various dispensaries and collectives—as my state refers to medical marijuana stores—and find that the budtenders in some stores really know their stuff, while others seem to be more like clerks than medical cannabis experts. If you prefer to have more guidance, I suggest visiting more than one store to get advice from more than one budtender.

You may be able to find a savvy doctor who is an expert on cannabis medicine who will advise you on the products and protocol that will be best for you. As I mentioned earlier, for some strange reason, in many jurisdictions the doctor who legally determines that you will medically benefit from cannabis is NOT allowed to advise you on product choices, potency, or dosage. Yet you may be able to find a doctor who does NOT write recommendations or "prescriptions" for cannabis but legally can—and does—advise patients on how to use the stuff. Right now, those doctors are still few and far between but, thankfully, their number is growing. An Internet search for a doctor in your area—or perhaps one at a distance who will work with you by phone or Skype—could lead you to one who is a perfect fit.

So how do you make protocol decisions when there's no one to guide you? When a trusted doctor gives us specific guidance, prescriptions, and treatment plans, it's easy to follow the directions we've been given. But, for the foreseeable future, most of us have to make our own determination on the medical cannabis protocol that's best for us. We have no choice but to fine-tune the dosage—tweaking and experimenting until we find the amount and frequency that is best. Then, depending on the protocol that's decided upon, some people may need to rapidly increase their dosage over a period of days or weeks in order to get the maximum benefit. As you peruse the many medical cannabis products available, you may find that there are several different types that would work equally well for you. If that's the case, you can focus on factors such as convenience, ease of administration, and price. Or, like many patients, you might decide to use multiple products simultaneously. They may be similar in strain—or you may find more symptom relief from totally different strains.

In a way, the fact that many patients need to take an active role in choosing their own products, dosage, and protocol may be good— because making these decisions requires that we tune into our own unique needs on a deeper level than usual. Each person has a different tolerance level, which is affected by their own unique body chemistry. For some patients a tiny amount of cannabis will provide the desired results, while others require a much larger dose to get a similar result.

A factor that's used to determine the optimum dosage of some medications is the patient's body weight. Yet, even though it seems logical that a person who is more than three times the weight of another person would need *more* cannabis to get a dosage that's right for him, that's not always the case. As an example, Rick Simpson shares a story about a 300-pound man and his 80-pound wife. When both of them took the same amount of cannabis, the wife was totally unaffected by it, while the husband became extremely stoned.

We don't know why some people are much more sensitive to cannabis than others or why some of them actually receive more benefit from lower doses. While it's a great idea to take all of the guidance you can get on dosage, there's still a lot of trial and error involved in determining the right dose. And, in most cases, as tolerance develops, you need to continue to titrate your dose.

A friend who is a medical cannabis patient told me that she had switched from taking lozenges made with cannabis oil (also called Simpson Oil) and was back on the lower potency capsules of whole cannabis extract that she had taken in the past. She made the switch because she was waking up groggy in the mornings and felt the oil was too potent for her. I was happy that she was figuring out the form, potency, and dosage that worked best for her. But then she said something that concerned me, "Of course, since the capsules aren't as potent as the oil, I'm no longer getting as much healing benefit." She had assumed that she had to take the higher-potency oil to get a therapeutic dose—and that a product that wasn't as potent wouldn't give her as much symptom relief. I explained that some experts believe that a "therapeutic dose"—the dose that would be the MOST effective for her—might be a small dose of a low potency product. Each person's body is different. There are no rules. Even a small dose of cannabis activates the endocannabinoid system. However, while some experts suggest that small doses can be the most therapeutic, others believe that you *can* take too little but it's difficult to take too much.

Knowing how important it is to have a positive attitude about anything that we ingest, I did not want my friend to feel that the healing potential of *any* cannabis product was limited. We just don't know what will work for any individual patient until they try it. Some people are highly sensitive to cannabis and do well at a dosage that's much lower than that used by most people. For example, one medical doctor told me he has a patient who took relatively low-dose extract capsules and achieved amazing progress in the healing of non-Hodgkin's lymphoma.

So what's the best way to decide on your medical cannabis protocol? Unless you have a trusted advisor to guide you, you will undoubtedly do what most people do—research your options as much as possible and then use your intellect to make decisions. That's what doctors do, after all. Yes, of course, doctors have a vast medical education. They also have knowledge of your symptoms and overall condition, as well as the results of any diagnostic tests you have taken. However, sometimes doctors are faced with the dilemma of two or more treatment options that are considered equally viable for the patient—and they must decide which one to pursue. In most cases, doctors probably *think* they are making the most educated choice—but is it possible that the really good ones may be tapping into their intuition or their "inner knowing" to a greater extent than they are aware? Having studied books and articles by many of today's leading edge physicians, I believe if they were asked about this most of them would respond with a resounding chorus of "Yes, that happens all the time."

I'm sharing this perspective on intuition here because I believe that most of us tune in to this "inner knowing" much more than we're aware of—and I believe it really serves us to do so. More and more research on intuition shows how critical tapping into it can be, especially when an "inner knowing" directs us on a path we wouldn't logically follow. Stories abound about professionals such as police officers and firefighters who have saved their own lives and the lives of others by following their "hunches." And the same is true for health professionals, who sometimes follow a hunch that doesn't make sense. Sometimes they order a medical test or prescribe a medication that isn't a logical choice but turns out to be the best decision they could make—and sometimes that "illogical" choice makes the difference between life and death.

Your Body's Internal Biofeedback Response System

A growing trend for a number of decades, especially among alternative health practitioners, is to decide among treatment and dosage options through diagnostic methods that tap into the patient's own internal biofeedback response system. There are several different ways to do this; however, they are all based on the concept that anything that is strengthening to your mind-body will give you a "positive/yes" response, while that which is weakening will cause a "negative/no" response.

It's possible that you have visited a doctor or other health practitioner who used one of these methods to determine which supplements or medications would be most beneficial for you, as well as how many you should take and how often you should take them.

Some doctors use high-tech electronic equipment to get these biofeedback responses from your body through electronic sensors that have been placed on your fingertips or other areas of the body, while others use low-tech methods that require no equipment. Whether equipment is involved or not, the goal of this type of biofeedback response system is to give practitioners a method to get "answers" directly from your body to determine the treatment options that are positive and beneficial for it.

The most commonly used biofeedback response method is a low-tech system that is referred to as *muscle testing* by most people. I've coauthored several books with Jerry V. Teplitz, J.D., PhD, an expert on this subject, who calls it *muscle checking*. Dr. Teplitz prefers the term *muscle checking* rather than *muscle testing* because the word "test" is a weakening, negative word for most people. Think about it—does being "tested" feel good to you? We've got so much baggage around that word that it can introduce a negative energy in the body before we even begin—and that could potentially impact the results we get *from* the body. So I prefer Dr. Teplitz's term *muscle checking*, instead of muscle testing.

Muscle checking usually requires a second person who does the checking procedure with you. However, there are also self-checking methods that you can do by yourself. I use self-checking frequently to get feedback from my body on whether to take a supplement or not. If the answer on a specific supplement is "yes," meaning that my body is conducive to the supplement, I do further self-checking to determine the quantity and frequency of the dosage.

Another biofeedback response method, called noticing, is more subtle. With noticing, you learn to determine which feelings and sensations in your body give you a "yes" or affirmative response—and which feelings and sensations give you a "no" or negative response. It takes a bit of practice for most people to tap into their body's own unique response system using noticing but, ultimately, it's worth the effort.

But, unless you follow a few important rules, the "results" you get may be skewed. To learn more about these biofeedback response methods, check out the demonstrations in Dr. Teplitz's free online video at http://Teplitz-inc.com/jte/SOSSelfCheck.wmv. There's also lots of fascinating information on ways to empower the body-mind on Dr. Teplitz's website at http://Teplitz.com. On this subject, I also recommend the pioneering work and books of Dr. John Diamond, as well as the work of Dr. Paul Dennison and Gail Dennison and the organization they founded, Brain Gym International (also known as the Educational Kinesiology Foundation) at http://BrainGym.org.

It's easy to learn to use internal biofeedback response methods. There are numerous ways to apply them in daily life—and they are always available when you want to tune into your body's internal wisdom. After all, you take your body everywhere you go, so you can use self-checking or noticing anywhere and at any time.

How to Evaluate Cannabis Products for Your Needs

By now, I hope I've made it clear that there are no definitive guidelines on cannabis product choices and dosage for the most efficacy. It's advisable to have a cannabis-savvy health professional to guide you. If you don't, you will have to make your own decisions on what product to take, as well as how often and how much. Advice from budtenders, websites, books, or a knowledgeable friend can be helpful; however, as with all things in life, we must be savvy about whose advice to follow.

Most of us take medications for one purpose—symptom relief. In many situations, we don't expect these medications to actually heal us, we just expect them to make us feel better by relieving our symptoms to some extent. But some patients have found that cannabis does both—it relieves symptoms and it also heals. To achieve greater symptom relief—and the *potential* for more healing— many savvy patients experiment with a variety of products until they've found one or more that most effectively meet their needs.

The research on medical cannabis that's available today is the tip of the iceberg compared with what's on the horizon. Research scientists will continue to achieve new breakthroughs as we learn more and more about the benefits of the many chemicals in cannabis. And that will lead to the breeding of more new strains that are more beneficial for specific symptoms and conditions.

This book does not attempt to advise patients on the specific cannabis strain or product that would be best for specific health conditions. To do so would double or triple the size of this book and— with all of the continued research and new improved strains—it would also guarantee that it is out of date before it is even published.

I suggest that you do as much research as possible on the specific strains, potency, and type of cannabis products that are being used to treat your symptoms or health condition so you will know what your options are. As you do this research, it will be helpful to keep track of it by creating a list of the information that relates to your situation, with a brief note about the reasons why it might help. I think of this as a "wish list" because it will provide you with a range of different cannabis options.

You will probably not find a single product that matches *all* of the criteria you come up with; however, this list gives you a good starting point that will help you prioritize the qualities in cannabis that may be most efficacious for you. Keep records on all of the sources you consult so you can revisit the information at a later date if necessary. Believe me, with the various options that are available today, it can get complicated. I suggest that you create a chart similar to the one I share below, which provides an example of what might work for a patient with the noted symptoms.

Sample Chart

My Research on Cannabis Strains and Products

1. List your health conditions and/or symptoms; for example:
- Chronic Pain
- Muscle Spasms
- Sleep Problems

Note: You may be focused on one or more major symptoms or conditions. As you do your research, you may want to add to this list; for example, perhaps you realize that anxiety—or one of hundreds of other symptoms—should be added.

2. Your Research on Strains and Products.
Below is a short list with the type of notes I suggest; your list may be much longer. Since determining which cannabis medicine is right for an individual often involves trial and error at this point in time, a chart like this will help you keep information at your fingertips.

Strain or product	Reason	Notes	Source(s)
Indica (one of two common sub-species)	Good for pain relief and muscle relaxation. Indica is usually taken in the evening because of its relaxing qualities, but helpful during the day for some.	Many products do not indicate if they are of the sub-species indica or sativa because they are a hybrid of the two. Also see Chapter 6.	Website: http://www.medicaljane.com/2013/07/25/cannabis-indica-as-explained-by-medical-jane/
Cannabinol (CBN), one of the 80 to 100 cannabinoids	Good for pain; has sedative effects		http://steephilllab.com/cbn-a-sleeping-synergy/
CBD to THC Ratio.	3:1 ratio of CBD to THC suggested for pain, muscle spasms, and nervous system.		Dr. X, in personal phone call
Raw Cannabis Products	Raw cannabis oil capsules in a 30:1 CBDa to THCa ratio provides symptom relief without psychoactivity and the unique qualities of the "acid" form of cannabinoids.	Check on whether the acid form of cannabinoids is best for my symptoms. Also refer to the section, "Raw Cannabis," in Chapter 3.	http://www.cannabisinternational.org/

In your chart, you'll want to list viable research on any of the chemicals in cannabis that might be specifically helpful for you, such as the cannabinoid CBN which is the second entry in the chart above. And, in addition to the cannabinoids, don't forget the other categories of chemicals, terpenes, and flavonoids, which also contribute healing benefits and are sometimes listed in the chemical profile. Even though most of these chemicals will be found in much smaller quantity than either THC or CBD, remember that they work together in a synergistic way—also referred to as the entourage effect.

While every patient desires a strain of cannabis with the most efficacious ratio of chemicals for their needs, it's possible that two products that are labeled as having the same chemical makeup may give you different results. For example, as documented on the CNN show, *Weed,* a high-CBD product from Colorado seemed miraculous in its efficacy for a little girl named Charlotte, whose debilitating seizures were reduced dramatically when she took it. However, when she returned to her home in New Jersey and was given a high-CBD product that was supposed to be the same as the Colorado product, it did not work at all. Her life-threatening seizures returned and continued at full force until the family was again able to obtain the Colorado product. The chemicals listed on the packaging may have been exactly the same on these two high-CBD products; however, in addition to the CBD and any THC in the product, there are also hundreds of other chemicals in each strain, all of which have a role to play, no matter how miniscule it might be.

The chances that the two products would contain all of the same chemicals, in the same exact quantities, is slim to zero. While a complete chemical profile of both products would prove that point, the profiles of most cannabis products either do not include chemicals that are found in very small trace amounts or they list them as "non-quantifiable." However, even in tiny quantities, they may still be a part of the overall therapeutic qualities of the strain. While analogies always come up short, I'll try this one: Any baker will tell you that a biscuit recipe calls for only small amounts of salt and baking powder in comparison to the other ingredients; however, the tiny amounts of those specific ingredients are critical to the final product.

In addition to seeking out the one perfect product or strain of cannabis that will have the best chemical profile for you, another way to achieve your goal is to combine two or more products, taking them together or at different times of the day. For example, let's say your health professional or your research suggests that a 2:1 CBD to THC ratio is recommended for a condition or symptoms that you have, but there's currently no 2:1 product available. However, you have access to a product that is 3:1 CBD to TIIC. By taking that product along with a second product that is high in THC, you can get close to the 2:1 ratio that you're seeking. It involves a bit of math, but it's easily computed. Let's say the 3:1 CBD/THC product contains 15 mg. CBD and 5 mg. THC. And let's say the THC product that you planning to take with it contains almost *no* CBD. To get close to a 2:1 ratio, you'll need to take approximately 2.5 mg. of the high-THC product. Combined, you would then have about 15 mg. CBD and 7.5 mg. THC.

If you're taking a product that causes little to no psychoactivity, except in rare exceptions, it's likely that you won't have to be concerned about getting stoned. (Review the section on Chapter 19, "More on the Raw Cannabis Movement," for more on those rare exceptions.) But if the product contains more than a smidgen of THC, you must also factor in your tolerance level.

In his book, *Nature's Answer for Cancer*, Rick Simpson explains why a patient with lung cancer might benefit from taking cannabis oil in more than one form:

> ... different ways of administering the oil can be combined with no harmful side effects and indeed doing so can be of great benefit in some situations. For instance, if I had lung cancer, I could combine ingesting the oil with the use of

suppositories and I would also vaporize the oil so it could be inhaled directly into my lungs. Both oral ingestion and suppositories work well to treat lung cancer and vaporizing the oil can also be of benefit for those who suffer from this condition.[90]

Some protocols, such as Rick Simpson's protocol for cancer and other very serious illnesses, which follows, are designed to get patients on a very high dose as soon as possible. But not all experts agree; some doctors who work with cannabis patients do *not* believe that more is better. Instead, they recommend taking very small doses and not increasing them over time. One of the theories behind the "small dose" protocol is that small doses are better at stimulating and strengthening the body's endocannabinoid signaling abilities. When taken over time, the small doses eventually help the endocannabinoid system function in a more optimal fashion so it can kick in and return the body to greater well-being.

Yet another dosage recommendation from some doctors is to gradually increase the potency and/or doses until symptom relief is achieved. John H. Hicks, MD, author of *The Medicinal Power of Cannabis: Using a Natural Herb to Heal Arthritis, Nausea, Pain, and Other Ailments*, is a holistic doctor who works with cannabis patients. He suggests increasing your dosage gradually until you achieve symptom relief, staying at that level for three months, and then reducing your dosage to half of that amount as a maintenance dose. However, when he is treating patients with very serious conditions, Dr. Hicks says that the protocol may vary considerably— and he also told me about patients who have achieved amazing healing results with very small doses.[91] Again, each patient's body chemistry is different—and, like so many other medicines, what works for one may not work for others, even if they have the same diagnosis or similar symptoms. And, with so many different strains available, there are a lot of options to explore.

No matter what protocol you're using, unless you're taking a cannabis product that causes little to no psychoactivity or you have already built a tolerance to cannabis, start with very small doses. Then allow your tolerance to develop by slowly increasing your dosage.

Rick Simpson has become known for the protocol he popularized for treating cancer and other serious illnesses, which has led to numerous reports of healings. The Simpson protocol is to take 60 grams of cannabis oil over a period of 90 days, starting with a tiny amount and building the dosage gradually until the patient is taking one gram of oil a day. That's a lot of oil. I know someone who takes twice that amount of oil daily for health purposes and he does well on it, saying that morning tea gets rid of any grogginess he experiences. However, unless they have developed a high level of tolerance, patients who are taking a gram or more of cannabis oil a day may find that it is difficult to do anything other than rest and sleep. In fact, some patients on that much oil probably should not live alone as they may need someone to prepare meals and care for them. Remember, in most cases, this protocol is for patients with life-threatening conditions who need quick action and high quantities of cannabis. Some experts believe that patients with serious illnesses should take all they can, every way they can, of every available strain and product. Here's how Simpson explains it:

> It takes the average person about 90 days to ingest the full 60 gram treatment. I suggest that people start with three doses per day, about the size of a half a grain of short grained rice. A dose such as this would equal about ¼ of a drop. After four days at this dosage, most people are able to increase their doses by doubling the amount of their dose every four days.
>
> It takes the average person about 5 weeks to get to the point where they can ingest a gram per day. Once they reach this dosage they can continue at this rate until the cancer

disappears. By using this method it allows the body to build up its tolerance slowly, in fact, I have many reports from people who took the oil treatment and said they never got high. We all have different tolerances for any medication. Your size and body weight have little to do with your tolerance for hemp oil. Be aware when commencing treatment with hemp oil that it will lower your blood pressure, so if you are currently taking blood pressure medication, it is very likely that you will no longer need it.

When people are taking the oil, I like to see them stay within their comfort zone, but the truth is, the faster you take the oil the better the chance of surviving. At the end of their treatment most people continue taking the oil but at a much reduced rate. About one gram a month would be a good maintenance dose. I do not like to see people overdosing on the oil, but an overdose does no harm. The main side effect of this medication is sleep and rest which plays an important role in the healing process. Usually, within an hour or so of taking a dose, the oil is telling you to lay down and relax. Don't fight the sleepy feeling, just lay down and go with it. Usually within a month, the daytime tiredness associated with this treatment fades away but the patient continues to sleep very well at night.

The only time I would recommend that people start out with larger doses would be to get off addictive and dangerous pain medications. When people who are using such medications begin the oil treatment, they usually cut their pain medications in half. The object is to take enough oil to take care of the pain and to help the patient get off these dangerous pharmaceutical drugs. Taking the oil makes it much easier for the patient to get off these addictive chemicals.

I simply tell people the oil will do one of two things; it will either cure your cancer or in cases where it is too late to affect a cure, the oil will ease their way out and they can at least die with dignity.

Hemp oil has a very high success rate in the treatment of cancer. Unfortunately, many people who come to me have been badly damaged by the medical system with their chemo and radiation etc. The damage such treatments cause have a lasting effect and people who have suffered the effects of such treatments are the hardest to cure.

It should also be mentioned that the oil rejuvenates vital organs like the pancreas. Many diabetics who have taken the oil find that after about six weeks on the oil that they no longer require insulin since their pancreas is again doing its job.

Properly made hemp medicine is the greatest healer on this planet bar none. Once you experience what this medication can do you will understand why history and I call hemp medicine a cure all.

Treating Skin Cancer: If you can get some properly made oil, it will definitely work to cure skin cancer and usually it only takes a few grams of oil to accomplish the task. ... Apply the oil to the skin cancer and cover it with a bandage, apply fresh oil and a new bandage every 3 or 4 days and the cancer should soon disappear. I always tell people to continue treatment until the cancer is gone, then they should continue to treat the area for about two more weeks just as if the cancer was still there. Doing this will ensure that all the cancer cells are dead and I have never seen a cancer return if my instructions are followed. If you've had skin cancer for quite some time and the cancer is well established, it may take some time to cure. But usually even in quite severe cases the cancer will disappear in less than three weeks. In an extreme case it may take longer but if so, then just keep up the treatment until it is gone. Many people can cure their skin cancer in no time, but it all depends on your own rate of healing and how deeply embedded the cancer has become.[92]

At times, I have followed a protocol that includes taking two or more different types of cannabis products on the same day. A mix of products works well for many patients and having multiple options allows us to fine-tune our needs. That may involve taking two products at the same time or taking different products at different times of the day. Healing is very individual—and you may need a lot less or a lot more cannabis or a totally different product than someone else to get similar results. I have a friend who has found that a low potency dosage works wonders for her. She is currently taking one-third of a low potency capsule of cannabis extract (mixed with organic butter) before bedtime. The product is a hard-shelled capsule, which she freezes in order to slice into smaller pieces. Once the capsule is frozen, she cuts it into three relatively equal-sized pieces and ends up with three doses.

Because it's so individual, I can't advise you on how much cannabis to take. As you progress on your medical cannabis journey, it's important that you regularly consider whether you should adjust your dosage upward OR downward—or perhaps add another cannabis product to your regimen in order to get the maximum benefits that it can offer to your body.

Also, as I discussed in the section on the healing crisis in Chapter 14, your body may detox when you take cannabis medicine. Signs of detoxing could be old symptoms recurring or new or additional symptoms such as increased pain, pain you haven't experienced before, nausea, headaches, or insomnia. In these cases, if possible, while your body releases these toxins, it may be advisable to decrease your dosage a bit—and then gradually increase it again. If you can, consult a cannabis-savvy doctor or other medical cannabis expert to help make a determination like this.

Be Open to Adding New Cannabis Products to Your Regimen

As I mentioned in Chapter 1, when I started taking a new cannabis product that was high in CBD and extremely low in THC, a chronic cough that I've contended with for 25 years almost disappeared overnight. Since I'd been on cannabis for a year-and-a-half at that point in time, I was truly amazed that a different strain would make such a big difference—and do it so quickly. Before I started taking cannabis, my ever-constant search for relief unfolded a couple of nutritional supplements and another holistic treatment that collectively—over a number of years—brought improvement in the cough by about 50 percent[93]. But until the day I started on this new cannabis product the daily bouts of coughing were still a disrupting, energy-sapping, and challenging part of my life. The high-CBD cannabis didn't get rid of the cough altogether, but it has diminished by 90 to 95 percent in frequency and it is also much less severe.

It takes a long time for new medicinal strains to be developed, grown, and perfected. Until I got the high-CBD product that made such a difference, the high-CBD products that I tried didn't help with symptom relief. I'd often felt that the cough was probably connected to my overall condition and I was hopeful that it would improve as my overall health improves with cannabis. Even though my overall improvement has been gradual, even tiny improvements in pain management and energy levels can be awesome. But the improvement in my cough was a big surprise. When I first took that product, I wasn't even thinking about the cough and I certainly didn't expect it to just about go away—almost entirely—overnight.

Each person reacts a bit differently to each strain of cannabis—and what helps most people doesn't work for everyone. I encourage you to try new strains, new routes of administration, take more than one product if necessary, and titrate your dosage until you get the maximum results with each product. I now have my daytime cannabis and my nighttime cannabis and am grateful for all of it.

Patient Guidelines

- Keep a written log on which you record:
  - The exact product(s) you take
  - When you take it
  - How much you take
  - Any other details that seem pertinent
- Keep notes on how you respond to the product.
  - How long does it take before you feel a difference?
  - Do you feel a difference physically? Mentally? Spiritually?
  - What symptoms are improved: Pain, nausea, mood, flexibility, breathing, mobility, balance, mental fog?

Chapter 22

What Should You Tell Family, Friends, and the Kids about Cannabis Medicine?

When I first became a medical marijuana patient I was reticent to tell anyone. Despite the fact that my own trusted doctor encouraged me to try it and despite the symptom relief it was giving me, to be honest, it still felt icky. Sure, there were lots of stories in the media about patients receiving help from cannabis—and even patients who pronounced that they had been cured by it. But my head was full of a lifetime of stories about those who used the "evil weed," some of which were scary and threatening: arrests and long prison sentences; lives ruined; doctors, hospitals and government officials taking sick children away from parents who pursued this natural and proven healing wonder.

If you're a medical cannabis patient—or if you're considering becoming one—it's unlikely that everyone in your life will agree with that choice. Some of your family and friends are probably stuck in the decades-old stereotype and believe that cannabis is an "evil weed." They don't understand that medicinal cannabis is very different from back-alley "recreational" cannabis strains. The most important message you can impart to any family member or friend who is concerned about your use of cannabis is that you are knowledgeable about the subject and you are using it responsibly.

I understand why many people are still stuck in the numerous stereotypes about cannabis because I was one of those stuck people for a very long time. I was never opposed to medical cannabis but, for many years, its checkered history and quasi-legal status felt overwhelming. I simply didn't feel led to pursue it—until one day when I was desperate for a new option. Then, even after I started taking cannabis and experienced positive results, I was very guarded about whom I told. I've learned that it can be important to keep the specifics of our personal lives, and especially our medical care, close to the vest, so we're not put in the position of defending our choices to others. That's why, in the first month or so, only a few very supportive friends knew about "my new favorite herb," as I frequently refer to it. Then, as I found more and more improvement, I told more and more people. Now I'm telling LOTS of people, including you!

So who should you tell about your medical cannabis adventure?

Talking With Family and Friends about Medical Cannabis

In many cases, family and friends who are initially negative about cannabis become supportive when they learn the facts. But, until and unless they understand enough about it to feel good that you're taking it, it's natural that they may be concerned. Some people can probably be educated on this subject so they understand all of the many benefits it brings. Yet there may be a few people in your life who still believe that cannabis is an unproven medication—or who might be concerned that you may get high and do something stupid or dangerous. With a complex topic like cannabis, you can't expect everyone to support your decision right away. Those old concepts about *stoners* and *potheads* need to be uprooted bit by bit—and it may take a while.

I have a friend who loves to research the latest holistic health and nutrition information. In my social circle, he's on the leading edge when it comes to this stuff. When I told him that I was taking medical cannabis in capsule form and found it to be amazingly helpful, I expected him to be pleased and want to know more. Instead, I was stopped in my tracks by his negative reaction. That was surprising because it was not like my friend to be *un*interested in a natural product, especially one that had gotten so much positive attention in the media lately. I thought he might be interested if he had a better awareness of the unique qualities of this herb and *how healing* it can be. But, in talking a bit further, the information I shared still didn't seem to influence him. *Then* he mentioned his teenage son—and suddenly his response and lack of interest started to make sense. I realized that my friend's immediate response of skepticism was rooted in concern for his son's well-being; the stereotypes he held about cannabis initially kept him from wanting to explore it further. However, over time, because of all the benefits he knew I was experiencing from it, as well as more and more positive stories in the media, he became interested in knowing more. He even arranged a one-on-one lunch—just me and his son—in part so I could explain medical cannabis and how much it has helped me. And I also gave both father and son early drafts of this book so they could learn more.

Another friend also had very mixed feelings about medical cannabis. On one hand, she had heard great things about it and thought it might help with the chronic, debilitating pain she suffered. Yet, on the other hand, she was also stuck in the stereotypes about cannabis and felt embarrassment and shame for even thinking about it. Eventually, her desire for greater physical well-being trumped the shame and she became a medical cannabis patient—and was delighted with the pain relief and improved sleep she experienced.

The reactions from these two friends are typical of the ways people perceive medical cannabis.

If any of your family members or friends express concern about .your cannabis use, let them know that taking cannabis is, in many ways, similar to taking allopathic, pharmaceutical drugs, many of which have their own lists of precautions. Many common over-the-counter and prescription pharmaceutical drugs come with the U.S. government's Food and Drug Administration's mandated warnings, such as potential risks, adverse reactions, contraindications, and precautions, including the potential for negative interactions that can arise between drugs when we take more than one concurrently. Explain to your family and friends that many people who are suffering from the terrible side effects of prescription drugs could be helped considerably by this sacred herb.

I don't choose to spend much time on the subject of "why" the United States and many other governments around the world went off track on this awesome healing herb for most of a century. Are the profits of pharmaceutical companies more important than having safe and effective natural medicines like cannabis available to those who can benefit?

The lies about cannabis have had a negative impact on countless lives. The war on cannabis has been a big factor in keeping prison populations high for decades. And with many of the prisons in the U.S. now run by private companies, there are great profits being made when those cells are full. There are also parallels to other arenas in which society has allowed big business to make the rules. For example, food industry executives will tell you that they offer nutritious foods, even though many—if not most—of the processed foods on store shelves are filled with preservatives, additives, genetically modified organisms, bovine growth hormones, antibiotics, hydrogenated trans-fat oils, low-quality sweeteners, so-called "natural" flavors that are actually synthetic, laboratory-concocted food agents, and other low-quality ingredients.

My hope is that the stereotypes will fade and, in the very near future, every medical cannabis patient will feel comfortable telling anyone and everyone how much it has helped them, without concern for the reaction they might receive.

Talking with the Kids about Medical Cannabis

When it comes to children's safety, it makes sense to treat medical cannabis with the same respect as pharmaceutical drugs. *Keep all cannabis products in a safe, secure place where kids can't access them.*

Of course, there's one huge exception to the "cannabis isn't for kids" rule—and that's when a child is the medical cannabis patient. Reports of children, some of whom are quite young and quite ill, being helped and sometimes even healed by medical cannabis abound in the media and online. Dr. Sanjay Gupta reported an amazing healing story on CNN about a 3-year-old girl who suffered 300 seizures a week, each of which was so severe that it was potentially life threatening. After starting on a strain of high-CBD cannabis oil, this darling little girl's seizures went down to two a month. However, she was also given a different strain of high-CBD oil that did not help at all and her seizures returned full force. Then, thankfully, her parents were able to get more of the helpful high-CBD strain and, once again, her seizures decreased to about two a month. This experience is more evidence that each strain is almost like a different medicine.

Clearly, cannabis is a wonder herb that often seems almost miraculous—and its benefits can help people of all ages. In some cases, children who have been successfully treated with cannabis had previously been on pharmaceutical drugs that were very hard for their little bodies to deal with. When they are put on cannabis, instead of all of the negative side effects of those drugs, the hundreds of chemical compounds in cannabis promote balance and harmony to all of the body's systems. A medical cannabis expert who followed the case of an eight-year-old patient noted to me that the child had an impressive degree of tolerance and his experience of getting high was simply feeling sleepy. Of course, our desire is not to get these young patients high; therefore, when they are efficacious, the newer low-psychoactive and non-psychoactive medical cannabis products may be the best fit.

But whether the patient is a child or an adult, how do you tell the kids in your life that this so-called "drug," which has a long history of being illegal, is really a good, healing herb? And what about the teenagers? What do you tell teens and pre-teens about using something that they have been told is illegal and wrong? Will teens think that another person's use of medical cannabis is a permission slip for them to use it illegally?

The following excerpt from the book, *Marijuana is Safer: So Why Are We Driving People to Drink?* by Steve Fox, Paul Armentano, and Mason Tvert, gives some perspectives that should bring some relief to parents on this subject:

> ...implementing legal yet restricted access to cannabis is not necessarily associated with increased marijuana consumption among young people. (To repeat, marijuana use by young people *fell* in California following the enactment of laws allowing for the sale of cannabis to qualified adults.) Let us explain why we believe this is the case. One, even under our current system of criminal marijuana prohibition, almost 90 percent of teenagers report on government surveys that marijuana is easy to get. In fact, many high school surveys indicate that teens can more readily purchase illicit cannabis than buy alcohol or tobacco, both of which are legally available to adults but cannot be sold to children. One study

by the National Center on Addiction and Substance Abuse (CASA) even reported that 23 percent of teens said that they could buy pot in an hour or less. That means nearly a quarter of all teens can already get marijuana about as easily—and as quickly—as a Domino's pizza! In truth, no system we can think of could possibly provide our children with greater access to cannabis than the system we already have in place: prohibition.

That said, we are not going to deny that some young people will still gain access to marijuana under a regulated system, just as some young people today have access to alcohol. Of course those who do will be obtaining a regulated product of known quality that is sold from a state-licensed retail outlet. This scenario, while hardly ideal, is still far better than the situation that exists today where millions of children are purchasing an unregulated product of unknown quality from millions of unlicensed sellers who have a financial incentive to encourage their customers to use other illegal substances like cocaine or methamphetamine. And don't forget, under our current system of prohibition teens don't even need to possess a fake ID to buy pot.

Truth be told, however, we do not assume that most teens, or even a strong majority of young people, will suddenly crave marijuana if it were legally available for adults. Virtually every teenager can already get his or her hands on cannabis now if he or she chooses. Yet it is apparent that most young people who quit using marijuana, or that never use it in the first place, abstain from it *despite* possessing the means to readily obtain it.[94]

Another article, "How Legalizing Marijuana Is 'Safer for the Children'" by Jeandre Gerber, also concludes that kids who have legal access to cannabis may be less likely to use it:

Portugal and several other countries decriminalized drugs and found that roughly a decade later less children were consuming drugs. Strangely it seemed that even when drugs were more available there was less desire from the youth to consume it. With an open approach to drug use the health care system adapted and less people overdosed and the addiction rates declined. When marijuana becomes "normal" kids will not covet it as much as they currently do.[95]

Chapter 23

What about Legal Issues, the Workplace, Travel, and Driving?

In this chapter we'll address some of the more pesky and troublesome issues for medical cannabis patients.

Legal Issues

As the public becomes more and more accepting of this awesome herb, legal use of cannabis for medical purposes is becoming more and more commonplace—and in some places cannabis is now legal for recreational purposes as well. However, as long as the U.S. government continues to unjustly and unscientifically list cannabis as a Schedule I drug, being a patient with a legal medical marijuana designation doesn't mean that you can take cannabis with impunity. And, of course, there are many countries where cannabis use is still totally illegal and carries stiff criminal penalties.

As a medical cannabis patient, it's a good idea to keep up with any changes in the law in your part of the world. If you have any concerns about local laws or family law issues, knowing your medical cannabis rights can be vitally important. For example, I have heard numerous stories of medical marijuana patients who lost custody of their children despite the fact that they were legally using the herb. Laws are changing quickly; don't assume anything. If you live in the U.S., the Procon.org website includes a summary of each state's laws at http://medicalmarijuana.procon.org/view.reszource.php?resourceID =000881. If you need any legal advice on medical cannabis issues, your local dispensary or collective may be able to refer you to an attorney who is an expert on the medical cannabis laws in your state or jurisdiction.

Despite the growing acceptance of cannabis in many parts of the world, it may take quite a while before it's universally appreciated again, as it was throughout most of history. With so many people still stuck in the decades-old negative stereotypes about cannabis, common sense dictates that you be discrete when you use it. It's simply not necessary for the people around you to know that you use medical cannabis unless you want them to know. Of course, it's a bit easier to keep your cannabis use confidential if you don't have its very obvious odor lingering on your hair or your clothes. Edibles or capsules or oil in a syringe may leave you with a bit of "cannabis-breath," but they don't cause the same degree of odor as smoking or using a pipe or bong. And vaporizers like the newer battery-operated vape-pens, which look like e-cigarettes, provide an odorless option as well.

The Workplace

How about the workplace? Can you be a medical cannabis patient and hold down a job? Most patients say medical cannabis doesn't interfere with their jobs. In fact, many believe that they are *more* productive, creative, relaxed, and energized *because* they take medical cannabis.

Should you tell your boss or coworkers about your wonderful new medication? Just because you've jumped through the hoops and now have legal access to medical marijuana in your state or jurisdiction, don't assume that those you work with or for will be okay with it. I suggest that you think twice before telling anyone at work– because you may open the door to challenges you aren't ready for. My hope is that this attitude about medical cannabis will change in the near future, but until it does, you may not want to share information with others that could threaten your livelihood.

So what happens when a patient's legal use of cannabis is *not* okay with their employer—or a potential employer? Again, this is an area where change seems inevitable. After all, many patients hold down jobs while taking medications. Medical cannabis is not the only medication that can cause physical impairment; there are *many* over-the-counter and prescription drugs that list physical impairment as a potential side effect. There's no reason that the superlative medication called cannabis should not be allowed by employers as long as patients use it responsibly. In that way, it's no different from many prescription drugs that other employees use.

In most places in the world, being a "legal" cannabis user does not guarantee that you will be allowed to *get* or *keep* a job. A random— but required—drug test could lead to the disqualification of an excellent candidate or get a person fired in short order. An online article, "Protecting Patients in the Workplace," shared the fears and frustrations that workers shared with California NORML, a branch of the national marijuana advocacy group NORML:

> California NORML regularly receives calls from frantic workers in danger of job loss. Ironically, many tell us that it's marijuana that enables them to be productive workers by managing their pain without opiates, or allowing them to sleep, or staving off migraine headaches. But unless they can

stomach pharmaceutical medications for their ailments, they're out of luck when it comes to the job market.[96]

The NORML article continues with a clever and obvious point on the subject of job security for medical marijuana patients from California State Senator Mark Leno: "I'm a fierce champion of the reasonable," joked Sen. Mark Leno .... "I don't think the voters of California, when they passed Prop. 215, intended it to only benefit unemployed people."[97]

If you are job hunting and face the possibility of a drug test when applying for a job—or if your current employer does random tests for illegal drugs—you may have to face the issue head-on. In order to clear the body of all traces of cannabis, one option is to quit taking it and go on a detoxification cleansing program, such as a detox tea. However, the length of time required to cleanse your body of any traces of cannabis varies considerably from person to person. Even if you stop taking cannabis for several weeks, it still may be possible for a drug test to identify the herb's metabolites or waste products in your body. An Internet search on "marijuana detox" will help you find the best options; however, be cautious and savvy as you proceed.

As time goes by, this conflict will get sorted out and our rights as patients will, I believe, triumph. I look forward to the day when employers understand that the presence of cannabis metabolites in your system does not mean that you're impaired. From my perspective, the bottom line for employers is to have a workforce that is productive, happy, and healthy. Perhaps, over time, some of them will understand that employees who use medical cannabis are pursuing a holistic path to healing and wellness that might make them, overall, *better* at their jobs, especially when compared to those who use conventional allopathic treatments that cause negative side effects. My hope is that a new paradigm will lead to enlightened business owners who are progressive on this subject. At that point, hopefully, medical cannabis will regain its rightful position in *everyone's* medicine cabinet—or just about everyone's, anyway.

Travel

As someone who has been helped so much by cannabis, I definitely want to be able to take it with me when I travel. Yet, on the other hand, nothing is worth the possibility of being arrested because of this herb. Therefore, it's obvious that we all need to know the laws about the use of cannabis in the places where we travel—and use extreme caution when traveling to a state or country that doesn't allow it to be used medically.

The first time I traveled out of state after I started taking cannabis, I was very nervous about taking it along. Even though I can legally use cannabis in my own state, with such ambiguous laws around the country and around the world, there were no guarantees that I would be immune to prosecution if it was found in my bags. I wanted to feel good on my trip—and nothing else has even come close to helping me get as good a night's sleep as my nightly cannabis regimen. But I kept thinking about the drug-sniffing dogs I'd seen checking carry-on bags at airports—and those thoughts gave me a lot of concern because the cannabis medicine I was taking at the time *definitely* smelled like cannabis.

I decided to take cannabis capsules that have a very low THC content and look like vitamin E capsules. I packed the precious capsules along with my other supplements in a zippered plastic bag, then put that bag into another plastic bag, and prayed that my plan would work. Luckily I made it there and back home again. I was able to take my cannabis on my trip—and no one seemed to be the wiser. But that doesn't mean I'm recommending my method to you. Each person has to do whatever feels right and whatever feels safe.

I was extremely grateful that these capsules gave me the symptom relief I needed to sleep at night—even though it was a totally different product from those I was using on a daily basis at home. To me, the most intriguing thing is that I can switch the type and form of cannabis I take, as well as the potency and quantity, and still get results. That may not be the case for all patients, but that's been my experience.

Whether you are traveling in your home area—where medical use of cannabis is (hopefully) legal—or to another part of your country or the world, be sure to carry your medical marijuana paperwork with you. And, when you're traveling by car, it's a good idea to carry your cannabis in the trunk. That way, if you happen to get into an accident or if you are stopped by the police for any reason, at least you won't have the cannabis on your person. (However, don't put cannabis in the trunk if the weather is hot; it keeps better in a cool environment.)

Driving

It is not legal to drive or operate heavy equipment while impaired or intoxicated by alcohol, legal drugs, or illegal drugs. Unless you're taking a non-psychoactive form of cannabis, when you're "high," you're considered to be intoxicated. The high that you experience could cause some hallucinogenic and sedative effects, impair cognition and memory, and/or impact your motor skills and coordination. When I'm taking a form of cannabis that causes psychoactivity, I always allow at least eight hours from the time I ingest it until I have to drive. If I don't have that amount of time, I don't take the cannabis OR I take a non-psychoactive cannabis product.

One of the challenges for law enforcement is that there's not a universally accepted way to determine whether a person is high on cannabis. Because of controversies in the scientific community on how to set standards to detect if a driver is stoned, the laws in most medical cannabis states use vague language for what "impairment" means when it comes to cannabis. One exception is the State of Washington which includes specific wording in its law—if THC is present in a driver's saliva in a quantity of more than 5 nanograms per milliliter, that driver is considered impaired, regardless of whether there is any other evidence of the impairment.

The good news is that there is evidence that cannabis is *less of a problem* in driving safety in states that have legalized medical marijuana. In fact, after medical marijuana was legalized in 16 states and the District of Columbia, the number of fatal car wrecks *dropped by an average of nine percent* according to a recent study based on government data from the National Household Survey on Drug Use and Health and the National Highway Traffic Safety Administration. A *Time* magazine article on that study, entitled "Why Medical Marijuana Laws Reduce Traffic Deaths" by Maia Szalavitz, summarized the study. Here are some of the pertinent findings:

- The reduction in traffic deaths was comparable to when the national minimum age for drinking was raised to 21.
- Teen marijuana smoking did NOT increase in states that legalized medical marijuana.
- Although there was a rise in marijuana smoking by young adults in their 20s in those states, there was a simultaneous *reduction* in alcohol use by that demographic.
- And, to quote from the article, "... driving high is much safer than driving drunk. Research on stoned driving is inconsistent, with some studies finding impairment and others not; the alcohol data, however, is clear in establishing a link between drinking and significant deterioration in driving skills. The data also consistently shows that using both drugs together is worst of all.[98]

A study that's referenced in an article on CaNORML.org's website at http://www.canorml.org/healthfacts/drivingsafety.htm shows that drivers who have a small amount of THC in their system had a *lower* risk of being in an accident than drug-free drivers. Here's an excerpt from that article:

> In the largest U.S. survey of drug use and driving accidents to date, the National Highway Transportation Safety Administration found that alcohol was by far the "dominant problem." At the same time it found "no indication that marijuana by itself was a cause of fatal accidents." The report was delayed and not publicized because it failed to confirm the expectations of administration drug warriors.
>
> The NHTSA report did find that the combination of marijuana with alcohol and other drugs was highly dangerous. Similar results have been reported in other studies. For this reason, California NORML does not recommend permitting liquor sales on premises where marijuana is allowed.
>
> On the other hand, studies have found that marijuana by itself tends to be significantly less dangerous than alcohol. A second NHTSA study of marijuana on actual driving performance found that the effects of THC appeared "relatively small" and less than those of drunken driving. It found that marijuana appeared to produce greater caution in drivers, apparently because users were more aware of their state and ready to compensate for it, whereas alcohol tended to encourage speeding and risky behavior. However, it also noted that marijuana could be dangerous in emergency situations that put high demands on drivers, or in combination with other drugs, especially alcohol.
>
> Other studies have shown that at sufficiently high doses marijuana does impair driving safety. Lab studies have

demonstrated noticeable adverse effects for the first couple hours of intoxication, including impaired attention, unsteady lane control and following distance, and slower reaction time.

Most recently, a large-scale Australian accident survey found that drivers with higher THC blood levels—particularly those above 5 nanograms per milliliter (ng/ml) in plasma, indicating that the cannabis use had likely occurred within the past couple of hours were correlated with a higher accident risk. However, THC levels below 5 ng/ml were associated with a lower risk than drug-free drivers.[99]

Chapter 24

How to Deal With the New Normal—Being a Patient Requires Patience

A challenging health condition or serious injury can bring up a lot of fear. If it's a serious illness, we might wonder how and why the body succumbed to an invader that has seemingly "taken over" and now plays such a prominent role in our life. In the case of an injury, we may blame ourselves or others for causing it. In either case, any health challenge can be life-changing. We are forced to reassess our lives and our goals. Depending on the severity of the situation, we may need to make changes—big changes and small changes—in just about every arena of life as healing becomes our number one priority. As we renegotiate our responsibilities and commitments, we have no choice but to accept a "new normal" for as long as necessary.

I believe that almost any disease or health challenge can be healed or, at the very least, improved—and that includes those that are the result of genetic or developmental abnormalities. The body is programmed for wellness; therefore, in most cases something has gone awry or illness just couldn't have taken root. With a modicum of proper maintenance the body constantly compensates in every way possible to alleviate injuries, stresses, and diseases—and achieve homeostasis. But when the body is overwhelmed by too many challenges, dis-ease or injury can be the result. The immune system caves in to a cold or flu virus. Or a disc in the spine becomes irritated.

Or cancer cells, some of which are always present in the body but lying dormant, suddenly multiply and become our foe.

Illness is scary—and when the illness is serious or life-threatening, it can be totally overwhelming. It feels as if the body did battle with a challenger and the challenger won. As life takes us down a path we didn't plan to travel and certainly don't want to travel, we are confused and scared. But, if we want to get well again, we can't just ignore it. We must take the journey.

As I dealt with my own "new normal," my dilemma became: "How can I heal something that I—and my body—created without knowing *how* I created it in the first place?" Wearing another hat for just a moment, I'll share my perspective on this as a spiritual counselor. Some people look at an illness as an opportunity for spiritual growth and use the metaphor of "lessons" or "life lessons" to describe the experience that's unfolding. But the word "lessons" seems a bit harsh to me. The worldview that I prefer is that life—or my soul's agenda— has provided me with opportunities for constant expansion. Rather than seeing a health challenge as "something wrong" that's happened *to me*, what if it is very, very right and very, very wanted from my soul's point of view? Health challenges give us an amazing opportunity for spiritual expansion; it's an opportunity to let go of the status quo and press the "reset" button in our lives. And from my perspective, when we do that, we step into *more* of who we really are.

When a patient is given the news that he has a serious illness, his world is turned upside down. It's common to go into shock when we get this kind of news; however, some people have the "spiritual muscle" that's necessary to rebound more quickly than others. Those who do so tap into an inner clarity and determination that then fuels them and leads them to take inspired action. These are leading edge patients who understand that they must change many of the details and circumstances in their lives while they pursue possibilities and answers and solutions that feel plausible. And some of them achieve a spontaneous remission.

Dr. Joe Dispenza spent years researching the case studies of people who experienced spontaneous recoveries. While there was great divergence in the age, race, cultural and religious affiliations (if any), education, and financial well-being, these individuals shared some powerful beliefs that allowed them to align with body-mind healing, which were the common link among them. In his book, *Evolve Your Brain: The Science of Changing Your Mind*, Dr. Dispenza breaks these beliefs into four arenas, which I have excerpted below:

1. An Innate Higher Intelligence Gives Us Life and Can Heal the Body

The people I spoke with who experienced a spontaneous remission believed that a higher order or intelligence lived within him or her. Whether they called it their divine, spiritual, or subconscious mind, they accepted that an inner power was giving them life every moment, and that it knew more than they, as humans, could ever know. Furthermore, if they could just tap into this intelligence, they could direct it to start working for them...

2. Thoughts Are Real: Thoughts Directly Affect the Body

The way we think affects our body as well as our life... The people I interviewed not only shared this belief but also used it as a basis for making conscious changes in their own mind, body, and personal life...

3. We Can Reinvent Ourselves

Motivated as they were by serious illnesses both physical and mental, the people I interviewed realized that in thinking new thoughts, they had to go all the way. To become a changed person, they would have to rethink themselves into a new life...

4. We Are Capable of Paying Attention So Well That We Can Lose Track of Relative Space and Time

The people I interviewed knew that others before them had cured their own diseases, so they believed that healing was possible for them too... Each person had to reach a state of absolute decision, utter will, inner passion, and complete focus... These mavericks sat down every day and began to reinvent themselves. They made this more important than doing anything else, devoting every moment of their spare time to this effort. Everyone practiced becoming an objective observer of his or her old familiar thoughts. They refused to allow anything but their intentions to occupy their mind.[100]

When you step into a "new normal" with a desire for greater physical well-being, there's no choice—you MUST requalify your priorities. One of my favorite mottos is, "Life is subject to change." I make that statement a lot—especially when something seemingly goes awry. Rather than resisting or pushing against "what is," accepting whatever has unfolded—and seeing it as an opportunity—feels so much better to me. Change can be scary; but when we're able to tap into our own inner wisdom, we're able to open to new possibilities in our lives.

When your own physical well-being is your biggest priority, you may find yourself aware of your body in new ways. A fine-tuning takes place. This is the kind of fine-tuning that is selfishly driven because, to heal a dis-ease or injury, your body insists that its needs be met. And sometimes honoring these needs, which include reducing stress and allowing time for rest and rejuvenation, is more critically important than anything else you could do.

We've learned to push aside feelings so we can do what we need to do—work, school, childcare, laundry, meals, mowing the lawn, and the list goes on and on. Like most people, for my entire life I've pushed myself and pushed myself to do everything in front of me—everything that needed to be done. Or at least everything that I *thought* needed to be done. Out of necessity that has really changed for me in recent years. Most days, after getting up and ready to start my day, all dressed, with the bed made and a cup of coffee in my hand, I feel so exhausted that I need a nap. Pushing myself is fruitless when I lack the energy. Many times, the focus that is needed to write that email or return a phone call or put the dishes in the dishwasher takes more energy than I have available in the moment. I have had to let go of lots of things I love doing when my energy is limited.

As I discussed in earlier chapters, most of us are very good at shoving aside the feelings that don't feel good. In fact, we're experts at it. We've done it all of our lives. The most important question you can ask yourself when you are out of sorts is, "What emotion am I feeling right now?" and then really tap into your feelings and deeply *feel*. You can't uplevel a feeling of powerlessness or frustration or anger or guilt or fear by simply pretending that you're not feeling that feeling. Once you *own* the feeling in the moment, it is easier to move upward on the emotional scale to a better-feeling thought.

Good-feeling thoughts are healing; we know this because the body is flooded with positive chemicals when we feel good. Being okay with how you feel, both physically *and* emotionally, is important to the healing process. Resisting a health challenge, feeling bad about it, or taking on the role of a victim will only make it feel bigger and more challenging for you.

Here are some additional suggestions to consider as you step into a "new normal" that is positive, life-affirming, comforting and soothing:

- **Let go of victim/martyr energy.**
  While reaching for healing and greater wellness, it is critically important that we let go of the victim/martyr mindset. This mindset can easily creep up on you, especially when your health challenge feels overwhelming or when you don't feel well enough to do something you want to do. Every now and then I find myself sighing and realize that I have stepped into victim/martyr energy. I'm not talking about the kind of sigh that accompanies a heartwarming experience. The victim/martyr type of sigh is more like an extended "ahhhhh" that's offered in response to an unacceptable situation. Perhaps you occasionally do it too? Sometimes the sigh is low and soft as it comes out of us in an unconscious manner, even when no one else is around. And sometimes it's intentionally loud so everyone can hear it, like when a disgruntled shopper wants to show his disdain for the person ahead of him in line. When I hear someone else sigh like that, it's usually clear to me that they feel they are a victim of the circumstance they find themselves in. And when I find myself sighing, I acknowledge that I've slipped into victim energy—and I do whatever is necessary to shift my thoughts to a happier place.

- **Remember that you are worthy!**
  There's nothing you need to do to be worthy; you already are worthy. For many of us, our feelings of worthiness are directly correlated to how we show up in the world. We got the message at a young age that we have to be relevant or we're not important. My health issue has helped me come to a deeper inner peace about life. More and more, I am able to let go of needing to prove myself in any way. More and more, I simply rest in the spiritual awareness that the Universe always has my back—and there's nothing that I need to *be*, nothing I need to *do*, and nothing I need to prove to anyone to be a

valuable part of the world. I am valuable because I Am. And the same is true for you. Taking care of yourself first is the only way to rejuvenate.

- **Let go of the need to JADE—justify, argue, defend, or explain yourself.**
  Honor how you *really* feel in every moment. When we try to jump through hoops to please others we can create a lot of stress for ourselves. And, as we've all experienced, some people seem impossible to please, no matter what we do. If you are undergoing any type of treatment or therapy for a serious or chronic illness, healing is your first priority. If you have a job, a family to care for, and bills to pay, it's even more important that you honor your body first. Of course, that's not easy to do when we have responsibilities and chores that are vital to day-by-day existence. But remember, when traveling by plane, there's a very good reason that adults who are traveling with small children are instructed to put their own oxygen mask on first should an emergency arise—and then the child's. Clearly an adult who isn't breathing can be of no assistance to a child. And you, my dear reader, will be of no assistance to anyone if you aren't here or if you aren't well. So let go of caring what anyone else thinks and take care of yourself first.

- **Stop juggling so many balls and decide which priorities really matter.**
  When you become a patient, the "new normal" can feel like a juggling act. Patients who attempt to do everything they did before their illness while also pursuing healing are keeping lots of balls in the air. And that definitely adds to the feeling of being overwhelmed. The more you can let go of other people's expectations and follow your own inspired actions, the better.

That may mean reassessing your responsibilities to your family, your work, and your community to the point that you let go of some of those responsibilities—even some that you thought you *had* to keep. Most of us are dependable and trustworthy people and we often take on roles in life that other people expect us to continue fulfilling. We identify with those roles, we may get acknowledgement from others for doing them, and it can be comforting to do them. But, as you focus on healing, it may be necessary to renegotiate work, family and community responsibilities. There's a great deal of trust required when we reassess our priorities and let go of some of our commitments—and sometimes doing so is critical so the body can take the needed time to heal.

- **Be easy on yourself.**
  Since I've been a "patient," it's become common for me to forget to do something that needed to be done or to keep a commitment that I made to someone. Beating myself up about it doesn't help anything. In fact, it just makes me feel worse—and that's not conducive to healing. I believe that my Inner Being, which is what I often call my alignment *to* and connection *with* God, is always there for me, arranging life's myriad details and reminding me when I do need to do something by giving me a metaphorical tap on the shoulder. So, when I realize that I forgot to do something, I find the best way to think about it is that God has another plan for me. As I lean into this awareness more and more, fewer things seem to fall through the cracks—and more seeming miracles unfold on a daily basis. I sometimes forget that my Inner Being always has my back, but the more I drop my resistance and just allow God's love to support me, the better life is!

- **Distractions can help.**
Dealing with the constancy of symptoms is not easy. Cannabis has helped to quell my symptoms; however, even though the severity is less, they are, at this point in time, still present and still a challenge. I find that anything I can do to change my focus and distract myself helps. I suggest that you find distractions that help you to focus in a different direction. Any activity that requires focus may help with symptom management—watching a comedy-filled TV show or movie, preparing a favorite meal, or even cleaning out a drawer. A call to a friend may also be helpful in your quest to refocus. However, there are two cautions: 1) in most cases, it's better to *avoid* talking about your health; and 2) it's better if you avoid calling a friend who is a constant complainer.

- **Eat a super-nutritious diet.**
Our goal as patients should be to eat the most nutrition-packed diet possible to help the body heal. While there are lots of dietary guidelines available for patients based on specific health challenges, the most common recommendations from holistic practitioners include an alkaline diet, probiotics in the form of fermented vegetables and other probiotic products to reestablish the good bacteria that are so important to digestion and health, and high-quality water. I cannot overstress the importance of adding probiotics since most of us have consumed many antibiotics over the course of our lives, both through pharmaceuticals that we've been prescribed and through the food chain. These antibiotics have not just killed the "bad" bacteria in your gut; they do not discriminate, also killing the good bacteria that are important to our health.

    Many holistic practitioners believe that we become sick—at least in part—*because* the typical diet consumed in industrialized countries like the U.S. is very low in nutritive value, while it is also devoid of needed fiber and filled with some ingredients that are of questionable safety. (Did you know that many food additives and preservatives that are allowed in the U.S. are banned in European countries because they are considered to be unsafe?) Many of these doctors also blame the "typical modern diet" for toxicity in the body because they find that a majority of patients have decades of impacted waste hanging around on the walls of the intestines. Most people who eat low-quality diets don't even know that they are not properly eliminating waste—but, over time, this toxic build-up causes more and more problems for the body, which becomes less and less efficient in dealing with other invaders such as bacteria, viruses, etc. For this reason, some practitioners believe that it's critically important for patients to undergo a bowel detox or colon cleanse program as a part of a healing protocol, while others believe there are gentler ways to pursue the desired internal cleansing. Of the many leading edge, holistic voices on nutrition and health, I suggest starting with Dr. Joseph Mercola's http://Mercola.com, Dr. Andrew Weil's http://www.DrWeil.com, and Dr. Richard Schulze's http:/HerbDoc.com.

- **Indulge in vitamin P with every meal and snack.**
  When eating psychology pioneer Marc David talks about Vitamin P in his book *The Slow Down Diet*, he is focused on *pleasure*. And that's something any patient needs more of because feeling good is so important to healing. David shares revolutionary research that proves that the benefit the body receives from the food we eat is in direct proportion to the *pleasure* we get from eating it. Yes, you read that right. The more you *enjoy* every bite, the more nutrients your body absorbs from that food. Among the fascinating studies on this

topic is one that involved groups of Thai and Swedish women who ate the exact same meals. First, both groups ate a traditional Thai meal of rice, veggies, coconut, fish sauce, and hot chili paste. Then both groups were tested to see how much of the iron content from the meal was absorbed and they found that the Thai women had absorbed about twice as much. Then, both groups ate a typical Swedish meal of hamburger, mashed potatoes, and string beans, which had the same iron content as the Thai meal. But they had the exact opposite results. This time the Swedish women, who enjoyed their traditional dinner, absorbed twice as much iron as the Thai women. Then both groups were given the meals from their own country but the entire meal was put in a blender and turned into mush before being served. This time, even when eating foods they normally enjoy, the pleasure factor was obviously extremely low. Even though the nutritional content was exactly the same as the other meals, the women in both groups absorbed 70 percent less of the iron. David says:

> The inescapable conclusion is that the nutritional value of a food is not merely given in the nutrients it contains but is dependent upon the synergistic factors that help us absorb those nutrients. Remove vitamin P, pleasure, and the nutritional value of our food plummets. Add vitamin P and your meal is metabolically optimized. So if you're the kind of person who eats foods that are 'good for you' even though you don't like them, or if you think you can have a lousy diet and make up for it by eating a strange-tasting vitamin-fortified protein bar, or if you've simply banished pleasure because you don't have enough time to cook or find a sumptuous meal—

then you aren't doing yourself any nutritional favors. You're slamming shut the door on a key metabolic pathway.[101]

I wish everyone on the planet was able to tap into David's excellent, leading edge perspectives on this topic. Also, I want you to remember that you can also get Vitamin P in many ways within your daily life, not just from food, so I suggest that you milk it and savor pleasure *everywhere you can!*

- **Be sensitive to your energy level.**
  I have to constantly make decisions about my energy level and what my body can handle. When you are in the healing mode, that which you actually *have to do* can become very simple and very basic. **If your condition is acute**, your life may depend on how you handle your energy level because as much energy as possible needs to be available for healing; you don't have the extra energy for much else. **If your condition is chronic**, your enjoyment of life depends on how you handle your energy level. Getting enough rest is the most important priority in my life and it's a priority that I have to plan for. When I do too much, it often takes a couple of days of rest to get back to my "normal" energy level. There are many days when I don't have the energy to make my bed and I don't have the energy to return a call. And, most days, "cooking a meal" means heating up something that's in the freezer. I might decide to do some writing or simply respond to an email but find myself staring at the computer, unable to focus for more than two seconds on the words strung together on the screen in front of me. Other days, when my energy level is higher, I might be able to write for an entire hour or even two. There was a time when I loved shopping for and preparing a big meal. But over a period of time I realized that my body would

be really tired after a session in the kitchen, so I had to pull back from that kind of activity. I've also had to let go of some very basic ideas of being a good hostess. These days I rarely cook for my houseguests; instead, they often cook for me—or we order food in. Any activity that requires me to stand for a period of time is problematic, especially if I am overly tired to begin with. If I do too much, my body is usually extremely tired for a couple of days—and that often requires me to cancel other activities that I wanted to do. It's a balancing act. If I over-extend my energy level, I have a problem; but if I don't keep as active as possible, my body isn't happy either. For me, the "new normal" means many simple and fun activities are no longer possible, at least not in the same way I enjoyed them in the past, so I have had to evolve new ways to do things and adopt new rituals in my life. Keeping as active as possible, without overexerting, is an important balancing act for any patient.

- **Find ways to feel good and practice doing so as often as possible.**
  When you feel good emotionally, your body produces chemicals that enhance that state, so make it your intention to feel good as much as possible. When you are in any situation that doesn't feel good emotionally, whether it's a conversation with someone, a scene on a TV show or movie, or concerns you might have about another person, do whatever you need to do to step out of that situation. Become a savvy patient who cares more about her own well-being than anything else. That's the way we heal.

- **Treat yourself to more fun and joy.**
  Whether it's a movie, dinner with a long-time friend, or buying something on a whim, anything that uplevels your

happiness quotient is healing. Here's one of my examples: In the past, I rarely wore bracelets because I found them a bit bothersome, especially when I was working at a desk. But then I saw some bracelets on a friend's arm that had a lot of bling. They were shiny and sparkly and fun—and looking at them made me feel good. My friend told me where she got them, so, on a whim, I bought some of them in different colors. Since then, I wear them often—and when I look down at them, I smile and feel good. These bracelets represent feeling good to me. Do whatever you can to find touchstones that make you feel good and then tap into them as often as possible!

- **Be open and receptive to a miraculous healing.**
  I've heard numerous stories of amazing healings that had no explanation that made any sense other than that it was a miraculous occurrence. I suggest you keep an open mind and consider the idea that if other people can tap into a miraculous healing, you can too. It doesn't HAVE to take time. I personally know people who have been healed overnight of conditions that were considered life-threatening—and I've heard many similar stories from people I do not personally know. I also know others for whom healing took a bit of time but would still be considered miraculous, given the severity of their injuries or illness. After a traumatic brain injury, one friend was a quadriplegic; he was told there was no "hope" that he would ever move his limbs again. But he didn't agree. He "fired" his medical team and found hope through the power of his own mind. What unfolded was a "miraculous healing" that led to full use of his body and all of his limbs. On the topic of spontaneous healing, I recommend the websites, books, DVDs, research, and YouTube videos of leading edge doctors and scientists such as Joseph Mercola, DO; Andrew

Weil, MD; Larry Dossey, MD; Joe Dispenza, DC; Bruce Lipton, PhD; Mario Martinez, PsyD; Gabor Maté, MD; Christiane Northrup, MD; Lissa Rankin, MD; C. Norman Shealy, MD, PhD; John Sarno, MD; William Rader, MD; Norman Doidge, MD; Michael H. Moskowitz, MD; Marla Golden, DO; Paul Bach-y-rita, MD; Edward Taub, PhD; Moshe Feldenkrais, DSc; Anat Baniel; Lynne McTaggart; Gregg Braden; Dean Radin, PhD; John Diamond, MD; Caroline Myss, PhD; and Sue Morter, DC. Each of these experts share aspects of *how* and *why* spontaneous remission occurs.

For many patients, the "new normal" requires that we do a lot less of the stuff that used to be normal for us, while we shift into a spiritual and psychological place that is conducive to allowing the healing that we want. In this new paradigm, mind-body-spirit health is the biggest priority.

As I've said before, healing can come from many different sources. I must end with this. Even though it's obvious that I am a big advocate for cannabis medicine and believe it's a master herb that has helped many people to heal—sometimes from dire prognoses—there are many people on the planet who have found healing without it. Clearly, each individual's healing process is unique and I believe that success is more dependent on mind-body-spirit alignment than anything else. And that's why emotional healing is such an important part of the journey.

INDEX

Endnotes

[1] Nicoll, Roger A. and Bradley N. Alger; "The Brain's Own Marijuana," *Scientific American*; November 22, 2004, page 5; Accessed November 11, 2013, http://www.scientificamerican.com/article/the-brains-own-marijuana/

[2] "International Classification of Diseases 9 - CM 1996; Chronic Conditions Treated With Cannabis, Encountered Between 1990-2004," The American Alliance for Medical Cannabis, compiled by Tod H. Mikuriya, MD, Accessed June 15, 20014, http://www.letfreedomgrow.com/cmu/DrTodHMikuriya_list.htm

[3] Lipton, Bruce H., PhD, *The Biology of Belief* (Hay House, 2005) pages 53-54

[4] Gertsch, Jürg, Robert G. Pertwee, and Vincenzo Di Marzo, "Phytocannabinoids Beyond the *Cannabis* Plant—Do They Exist?", *British Journal of Pharmacology,* v. 160(3): June 2010, Accessed July 14, 2014, http://www.ncbi.nlm.nih.gov/pmc/articles/PMC2931553/

[5] Merriam-Webster.com, Accessed June 2, 2013; http://www.merriam-webster.com/dictionary/homeostasis

[6] "Hemp Facts," North American Industrial Hemp Council, Inc., Accessed October 12, 2013, http://naihc.org/hemp

[7] Eisenhower, Dwight D., Farewell Address to the Nation, television broadcast on January 17, 1961.

[8] "Cannabinoids as Antioxidants and Neuroprotectants," U.S. Government Patent # 6,630,507, Accessed July 1, 2014, http://patft.uspto.gov/netacgi/nph-Parser?Sect1=PTO1&Sect2=HITOFF&d=PALL&p=1&u=%2Fnetahtml%2FPTO%2Fsrchnum.htm&r=1&f=G&l=50&s1=6630507.PN.&OS=PN/6630507&RS=PN/6630507

[9] *Ibid.*

[10] Gupta, Sanjay, MD, "Why I Changed My Mind on Weed," on www.CNN.com, August 9, 2013, Accessed October 23, 2013, http://edition.cnn.com/2013/08/08/health/gupta-changed-mind-marijuana/index.html

[11] Grinspoon, Lester, MD, "Marijuana as Wonder Drug," Boston Globe, March 1, 2007, Accessed December 14, 2013, http://www.boston.com/news/globe/editorial_opinion/oped/articles/2007/03/01/marijuana_as_wonder_drug/

[12] "The Science of Cannabis," Canna-Centers, Accessed October 29, 2013, http://www.canna-centers.com/dr-tods-list

[13] "Man Cured of Cancer After Applying Cannabis Oil," Accessed July 18, 2014, http://www.youtube.com/watch?v=IYJyCgM8-_w

[14] Personal correspondence with Patrick Lang, September 30, 2014. Lang is a principle in the patients association, CA Provider, which can be accessed at http://MyCAprovider.com.

[15] Grinspoon, Lester, MD, "Medical Marijuana: A Note of Caution," High Times, Accessed October 26, 2013, http://www.hightimes.com/read/medical-marijuana-note-caution

[16] *Ibid.*

[17] Badiner, Allan, "High on Health: CBD in the Food Supply," on the blog, Benefits to Raw Cannabis Juicing, Accessed December 20, 2013, http://40dayrawcannabisjuicechallenge.blogspot.com/2013/06/high

[18] "The Science of Cannabis: The Endocannabinoid System," Accessed June 20, 2014, http://canna-centers.com/cannabis-science

[19] Samuelson, Gary L., PhD, *The Science of Healing Revealed*, published by Gary Samuelson, 2009, page 7

[20] Hoye, David; Mary Ann Harrel; and Al Gray; *Cannabis Chemotherapy: The Science of Treating and Preventing Cancer with Concentrated*

Marijuana Medicine; 2013, pre-publication edition. Available as free download at http://cannabischemo.info

[21] Nicoll, Roger A. and Bradley N. Alger; "The Brain's Own Marijuana," *Scientific American*; November 22, 2004, page 5; Accessed November 11, 2013, http://www.scientificamerican.com/article/the-brains-own-marijuana/

[22] *Ibid.*

[23] *Ibid.*

[24] George, Helga, "What Is Anandamide?" Accessed November 11, 2013, http://www.wisegeek.com/what-is-anandamide

[25] Senese, Fred, "Anandamide," General Chemistry Online, Accessed November 11, 2013, http://antoine.frostburg.edu/chem/senese/101/features/anandamide

[26] *Ibid.*

[27] Teitelbaum, Ilana, "Thinking Outside the Box About Addiction," Accessed November 11, 2013, https://english.tau.ac.il/sites/default/files/media_server/TAU%20Review%202011-12.pdf

[28] Weil, Andrew, MD, *Health and Healing*, (Houghton Mifflin Company, 1988) page 97.

[29] *Ibid.*, pages 98-99 and 101.

[30] Mercola, Joseph, "Documentary: Pill Poppers," (film review) Accessed December 20, 2013, http://articles.mercola.com/sites/articles/archive/2013/07/27/pill-poppers.aspx

[31] Weil, page 97.

[32] Gupta, Sanjay, MD, CNN television series, "Sanjay Gupta, MD," first aired October 17, 2012.

[33] *Ibid.*

34 Bachhuber, Marcus A., MD; Brendan Saloner, PhD; Chinazo O. Cunningham, MD, MS; Colleen L. Barry, PhD, MPP, "Medical Cannabis Laws and Opioid Analgesic Overdose Mortality in the United States, 1999-2010," *JAMA Internal Medicine* formerly *Archives of Internal Medicine*, http://archinte.jamanetwork.com/article.aspx?articleid=1898878, August 23, 2014, Accessed September 18, 2014.

35 McTaggart, Lynne, "Natural Medicine Is a Human Rights Issue," Lynne McTaggart email newsletter dated November 21, 2013, Accessed November 21, 2013, http://lynnemctaggart.com/blog/247-natural-medicine-is-a-human-rights-issue

36 Mercola, Joseph, "Doctors Are The Third Leading Cause of Death in the US, Killing 225,000 People Every Year," Accessed June 20, 2014, http://articles.mercola.com/sites/articles/archive/2000/07/30/doctors-death-part-one.aspx

37 Personal correspondence with Patrick Lang, August 20, 2014.

38 Personal phone conversation with medical marijuana expert, June 3, 2013.

39 "What Is CBD?", Copyright 2015; Accessed September 10, 2015; https://www.projectcbd.org/what-cbd

40 "Cannabinoids as Percent of Total Sample Mass," Chart Copyright 2011, Steep Hill Labs, Inc. Reprinted with Permission. http://www.steephilllab.com.

41 Cannabinoid chart, Copyright 2011, Steep Hill Labs, Inc. Reprinted with Permission. http://www.steephilllab.com

42 "Phytocannabinoids, An Overview," Posted January 20, 2014, Accessed July 15, 2014, http://steephilllab.com/phytocannabinoids-an-overview/

43 Bello, Joan, "Benefits of Marijuana: Physical, Psychological, and Spiritual, (Author's website), Accessed May 15, 2014, http://www.benefitsofmarijuana.com/benefits.php

44 Bello, Joan, *The Benefits of Marijuana*, (Lifeservices Press, 2008) page 30

[45] *Ibid.*, page 35

[46] *Ibid.*, page 33

[47] I studied the Buteyko method with Jan Leuken at http://www.buteykola.com; there are also numerous videos on this method on YouTube. I first learned about Buteyko Breathing on Dr. Joseph Mercola's website at http://articles.mercola.com/sites/articles/archive/2013/11/24/buteyko-breathing.

[48] Bello, page 29

[49] Samuelson, pages 45-46

[50] Hoye

[51] "Understanding Basic Healing Principles of Natural Cure" on website, Shirley's Wellness Café, Accessed January 7, 2014, http://www.shirleys-wellness-cafe.com/naturalhealth/philo.aspx

[52] Bello, page 126; an abstract of the study is available at http://www.ncbi.nlm.nih.gov/pubmed/8121737

[53] Lipman, Frank, MD, "Adaptogens: Nature's Miracle Anti-stress and Fatigue Fighters," Accessed September 1, 2015, http://www.drfranklipman.com/adaptogens-natures-miracle-anti-stress-and-fatigue-fighters/

[54] Bello, page 129.

[55] *Cannabis Rising: The Key In The Lock. Your Health Your Future* (online video), Accessed December 2, 2013, http://www.youtube.com/watch?v=90fQss8OL9Q

[56] "Cannabis For Infant's Brain Tumor, Doctor Calls Child 'A Miracle Baby,'" Accessed January 3, 2014, http://www.huffingtonpost.com/2012/12/01/cannabis-for-infants-brai_n_2224898.html

[57] Maté, Gabor, MD; *When the Body Says No: Exploring the Stress-Disease Connection*, John Wiley & Sons, Inc., 2003; preface 2011; page xi.

[58] Rankin, Lissa, MD, *Heal Yourself: Mind Over Medicine with Lissa Rankin, MD* (PBS Television Special, August 29, 2013)

[59] Martinez, Mario, The Mind-Body Code: How the Mind Wounds and Heals the Body (CD album); Sounds True; 2009. (Note: Dr. Martinez's book, *The MindBody Code: How to Change the Beliefs that Limit Your Health, Longevity, and Success*, was released by Sounds True in 2014.)

[60] David, Marc, *The Slow Down Diet*, (Healing Arts Press, 2005) pages 124-125

[61] Courtney, William, MD, "Medical Marijuana Is Safe for Children," *U.S. News and World Report*, January 1, 2013, Accessed October 9, 2013, http://www.usnews.com/opinion/articles/2013/01/07/medical-marijuana-is-safe-for-children

[62] Hoye

[63] "Hemp Oil Hustlers: A Project CBD Special Report on Medical Marijuana Inc., HempMeds and Kannaway," Accessed November 9, 2014, http://www.projectcbd.org/news/hemp-oil-hustlers-a-project-cbd-special-report-on-medical-marijuana-inc-hempmeds-and-kannaway/

[64] "The Young Decision: DEA Administrative Law Judge Findings," The Family Council on Drug Awareness, Content Copyright 2000-2004; Accessed August 30, 2015, http://www.equalrights4all.org/fcda/judge.young.htm

[65] Hoye

[66] Hoye

[67] Holland, Julie, MD, et al., *The Pot Book*, (Park Street Press, 2010)) pages 352-353.

[68] Amen, Daniel, MD, *Unchain Your Brain*, (MindWorks Press, 2010) page 39.

[69] Brown, Brene, PhD, LMSW, *Daring Greatly* (Gotham Books, 2012) pages 137-139.

[70] "Student-faculty Research Suggests Oreos Can Be Compared to Drugs of Abuse in Lab Rats," *Connecticut College News*, October 15, 2013, Accessed December 2, 2013, http://www.conncoll.edu/news/news-archive/2013/student-faculty-research-suggests-oreos-can-be-compared-to-drugs-of-abuse-in-lab-rats.htm#.U6iJxbFcu24

[71] Doidge, Norman, MD, *The Brain's Way of Healing: Remarkable Discoveries and Recoveries from the Frontiers of Neuroplasticity,* (Viking, 2015), pages 29-30.

[72] Hoye

[73] Fife, Bruce, ND, *The Healing Crisis* (Piccadilly Books, Ltd., 2010) pages 25-27.

[74] "What is CBD?," Project CBD, Accessed March 1, 2015, http://www.projectcbd.org/about/introducing-cbd/

[75] Marczyk, Ron, "Worth Repeating: Marijuana and the Psychology of Optimal Experience," Accessed December 21, 2013 on blog, Toke Signals with Steve Elliot, http://tokesignals.com/worth-repeating-marijuana-and-the-psychology-of-optimal-experience-2/

[76] "Medical Cannabis Provides Dramatic Relief for Sufferers of Chronic Ailments, Israeli Study Finds," January 24, 2013, Accessed August 13, 2014, http://www.sciencedaily.com/releases/2013/01/130124123453.htm

[77] Bello, Joan, *The Yoga of Marijuana*, (Lifeservices Press, Inc., 2015) page 63.

[78] Bello, Joan, *The Benefits of Marijuana*, (Lifeservices Press, Inc., 2008) pages 35 to 41

[79] Baca, Ricardo, "Edibles' THC Claims Versus Lab Tests Reveal Big Discrepancies," March 9, 2014, Accessed June 1, 2014, http://www.thecannabist.co/2014/03/09/tests-show-thc-content-marijuana-edibles

[80] Simpson, page 37

[81] Simpson, page 16

[82] "Cannabis International Foundation," http://www.cannabisinternational.org/index.php, Accessed September 30, 2015.

[83] Personal correspondence with Rev. Dr. Kymron deCesare, Chief Research Officer of Steep Hill Lab, Inc., May 5, 2015.

[84] Dawson, Leanne, "Juicing Cannabis: The Potential Health Benefits of Treating Cannabis Like a Vegetable" on the blog, Benefits to Raw Cannabis Juicing, Accessed January 3, 2014, http://40dayrawcannabisjuicechallenge.blogspot.com/search?q=captured+these+molecules

[85] Personal correspondence with Rev. Dr. Kymron deCesare, Chief Research Officer of Steep Hill Lab, Inc., June 28, 2015.

[86] Personal correspondence with Rev. Dr. Kymron deCesare, Chief Research Officer of Steep Hill Lab, Inc., February 22, 2015.

[87] Marcu, Jahan, PhD, "How Safe is Your Vape Pen?" July 14, 2015, Accessed 9-1-15, https://www.projectcbd.org/article/how-safe-your-vape-pen

[88] Dowd, Maureen, "Don't Harsh Our Mellow, Dude," *The New York Times,* June 3, 2014, Accessed June 4, 2014, http://www.nytimes.com/2014/06/04/opinion/dowd-dont-harsh-our-mellow-dude.html?smid=tw-NYTimesDowd&seid=auto&_r=1

[89] 420 Motoco, "How to Dose Correctly Using Rick Simpson Concentrated Cannabis Oil," Accessed November 1, 2014, http://www.420magazine.com/forums/methods-use-rso-rick-simpson-oil/204363-how-dose

[90] Simpson, page 35

[91] Personal phone conversation with Dr. John Hicks, June, 2014

[92] Simpson, Rick, "Dosage Information" at http://www.PhoenixTears.ca, the official website of Rick Simpson; Accessed December 21, 2013, http://phoenixtears.ca/dosage

[93] The supplements that improved the cough were ASEA (a product sold via multi-level marketing) which supplies redox signaling molecules to the cells of the body, available at http://www.NormaEckroate.teamASEA.com; and Virxal, a type of high quality minerals called humic acid that's available online. I also credit the Buteyko Breathing method for even greater improvement in my ability to breathe more deeply. I studied the Buteyko method with Jan Leuken at http://www.buteykoLA.com; there are also numerous videos about it on YouTube. I first learned about Buteyko Breathing on Dr. Joseph Mercola's website at http://articles.mercola.com/sites/articles/archive/2013/11/24/buteyko-breathing

[94] Fox, Steve, Paul Armentano, and Mason Tvert, *Marijuana is Safer: So Why Are We Driving People to Drink?,* (Chelsea Green Publishing, 2009), pages 167-168.

[95] Gerber, Jeandre, "How Legalizing Marijuana Is 'Safer for the Children,'" at www.MarijuanaDoctors, Accessed 12-7-13 at https://www.marijuanadoctors.com/blog/medical-marijuana-research/How-legalizing-marijuana-is-Safer-for-the-children-

[96] Komp, Ellen, "Protecting Patients in the Workplace" from *The Daily Californian*, January 17, 2012, Accessed December 14, 2013, http://www.dailycal.org/2012/01/17/protecting-patients-in-the-workplace/

[97] *Ibid.*

[98] Szalavitz, Maia, "Why Medical Marijuana Laws Reduce Traffic Deaths, *Time Magazine*, December 2, 2011, Accessed December 14, 2013, http://healthland.time.com/2011/12/02/why-medical-marijuana-laws-reduce-traffic-deaths/

[99] Gieringer, Dale, PhD, "California NORML Research Report: Driving Studies Show Limited Accident Risk from Marijuana," Accessed December 30, 2013,
http://www.canorml.org/healthfacts/drivingsafety.htm

[100] Dispenza, Joe, *Evolve Your Brain: The Science of Changing Your Mind*, Health Communications, Inc., 2007, pages 39, 42, 47 and 51.

[101] David, Marc, *The Slow Down Diet*, Healing Arts Press, 2005, pages 103-104

About the Author

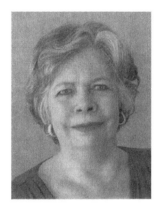

Norma Eckroate is a medical marijuana patient and a writer. She has co-authored numerous books, including the bestselling *The Natural Cat* with Anitra Frazier and *The Dog Whisperer* and *The Puppy Whisperer*, both written with Paul Owens. Eckroate has co-authored nine other books on a variety of topics, including three books with stress management and brain optimization expert, Dr. Jerry V. Teplitz: *Switched-On Living*, *Switched-On Selling*, and *Switched-On Networking*. She became a licensed spiritual practitioner at the Agape International Spiritual Center in 2001 and has also worked extensively in theatre and television. Eckroate lives with her two cats in Los Angeles.

CPSIA information can be obtained
at www.ICGtesting.com
Printed in the USA
FSOW01n1215290116
16338FS